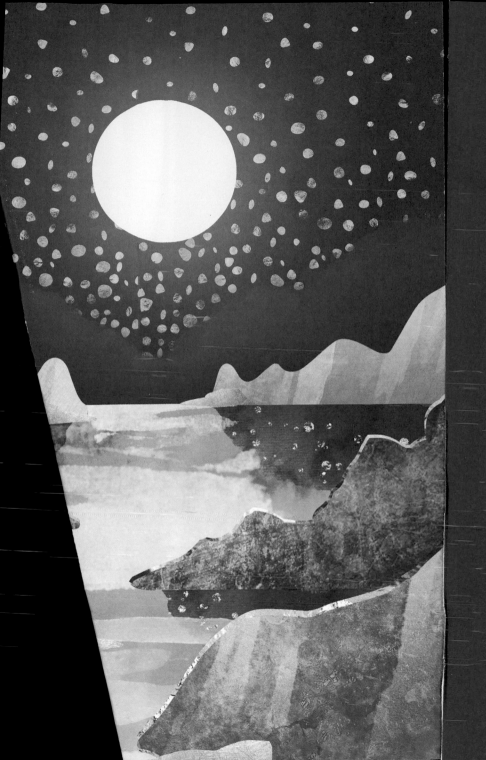

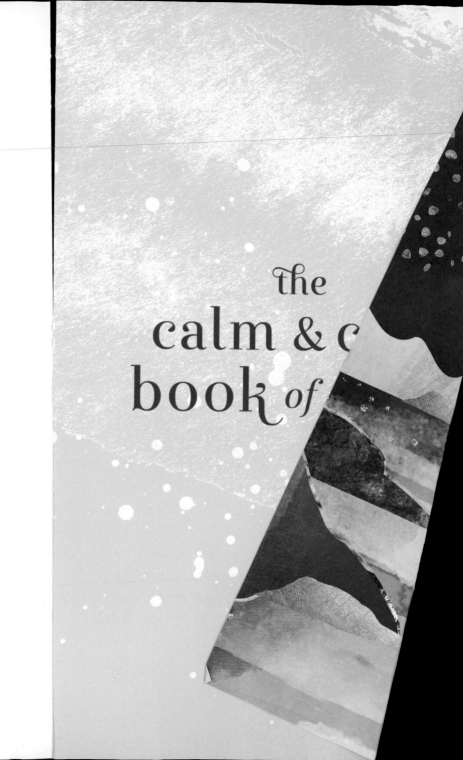

the
calm & c
book of

the
calm & cozy
book *of* sleep

Rest + Dream + Live

Beth Wyatt

ROCK
POINT

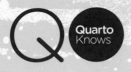

Brimming with creative inspiration, how-to projects, and useful information to enrich your everyday life, Quarto Knows is a favorite destination for those pursuing their interests and passions. Visit our site and dig deeper with our books into your area of interest: Quarto Creates, Quarto Cooks, Quarto Homes, Quarto Lives, Quarto Drives, Quarto Explores, Quarto Gifts, or Quarto Kids.

First published in 2020 by Rock Point, an imprint of The Quarto Group, 142 West 36th Street, 4th Floor, New York, NY 10018, USA
T (212) 779-4972 F (212) 779-6058
www. QuartoKnows.com

Rock Point titles are also available at discount for retail, wholesale, promotional and bulk purchase. For details, contact the Special Sales Manager by email at specialsales@quarto.com or by mail at The Quarto Group, Attn: Special Sales Manager, 100 Cummings Center Suite, 265D, Beverly, MA 01915, USA.

10 9 8 7 6 5 4 3 2

ISBN: 978-1-63106-687-0

Publisher: Rage Kindelsperger
Creative Director: Laura Drew
Managing Editor: Cara Donaldson
Senior Editor: Erin Canning
Cover Design: Laura Drew
Interior Design: Jen Cogliantry
Cover Illustration by @spacefrogdesigns
Interior illustrations pages 8-9, 18-19, 32-33, 46-47, 58-59, 72-73, 82-83, 96-97, 112-113, 123 by @spacefrogdesigns
Author Photo: Rae Connell

Library of Congress Cataloging-in-Publication Data

Names: Wyatt, Beth, author.
Title: The calm and cozy book of sleep : rest + dream + live / Beth Wyatt.
Description: New York : Rock Point, [2020] | Series: Live well | Summary:
    "The Calm and Cozy Book of Sleep is a down-to-earth guide with expert tips to get you to sleep and stay asleep"-- Provided by publisher.
Identifiers: LCCN 2020007157 (print) | LCCN 2020007158 (ebook) | ISBN 9781631066870 (hardcover) | ISBN 9780760367421 (ebook)
Subjects: LCSH: Sleep--Popular works. | Sleep disorders--Popular works.
Classification: LCC RA786 .W93 2020 (print) | LCC RA786 (ebook) | DDC 612.8/21--dc23
LC record available at https://lccn.loc.gov/2020007157
LC ebook record available at https://lccn.loc.gov/2020007158

Printed in China TT112020

For my grandmothers,
Dorothy and Marianne,
for passing down their stellar
catnapping genes.

Contents

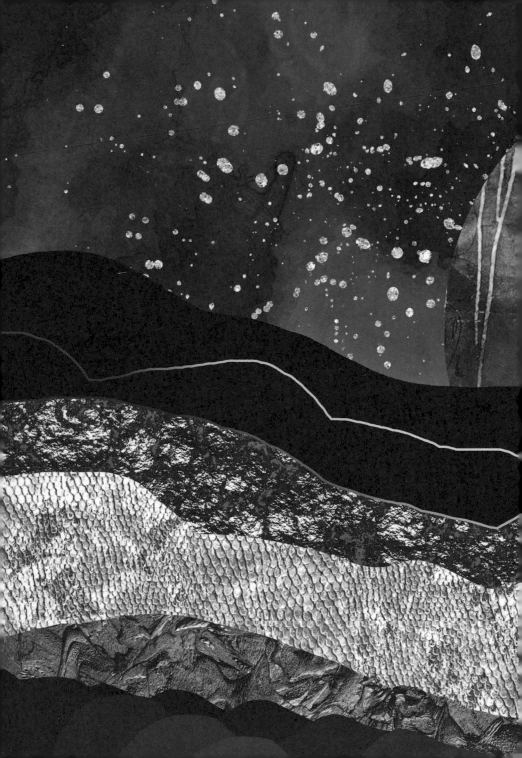

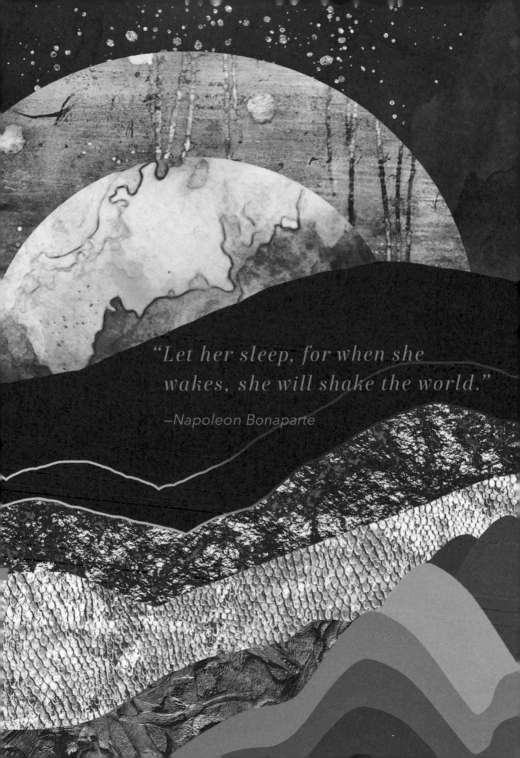

"Let her sleep, for when she wakes, she will shake the world."

—Napoleon Bonaparte

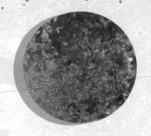

Introduction

HOW CHANGING MY SLEEP CHANGED MY LIFE

My relationship with sleep hasn't always been blissful. As a child, I enjoyed the bedtime-story portion of the night, but the getting-into-bed part cut into my valuable playtime. I don't remember much about my sleep as a teenager except for sneaking in the front door after midnight, sleeping in as late as possible every morning, and napping during class—meaning that my sleep habits were sketchy at best.

In my twenties and most of my thirties, I was too busy working on creative projects and binge-watching my favorite shows to sleep much. I proudly referred to myself as a night owl and delayed going to bed for as long as possible. When I was finally too exhausted to keep my eyes open, I would reluctantly fall into bed and then lie awake for hours, my mind racing with negative thoughts and anxiety. My brain's favorite topics were conversations I had had earlier that day that didn't end as I had hoped. Bedtime was my brain's chance to relive those conversations, so that I could make sure I won this time around. I also did a lot of pondering of deep topics, such as the meaning of life, how it would feel if my soul lived on for eternity, and how long you're supposed to wait before you unfollow your friend's recent ex on Facebook. When I finally did fall asleep, I was usually restless. If I woke up in the middle of the night, it was "game over" for me. Time to relive another conversation from my day or sing a song to the beat of the ticking clock on the wall.

I would refer to my sleep hygiene during those years as "just squeaking by." I was dragging myself through the day with no time to properly take care of myself. I was catching colds when everyone around me was sick and napping for hours in my free time. I was thirty years old when I realized my chronic pelvic pain was caused by hormonal imbalances, and I was diagnosed with polycystic ovarian syndrome and endometriosis. My weight was climbing and I didn't have the time or energy to do anything about it. I was spending money on a gym membership every month and filling my journal with good intentions of early morning workouts and healthy meal prep before work, but now I spent every possible minute in bed, trying desperately to catch up on missed sleep.

I believe I was a night owl for so long because being in bed was stressful for me. Why would I put aside whatever enjoyable project I was working on just to lie in bed wide awake, worrying about my soul in the afterlife?! I had better things to do, like crocheting a hat or watching episode after episode of *Arrested Development*.

Despite all of this, I was a happy person. I was in a healthy relationship and managed to find the fun in every situation, but I felt as if I was living in a fog. My desk job was torture because I couldn't focus long enough on any one project. I was fighting to stay awake, taking frequent breaks, and fantasizing about all the soft places in the room that would make for the perfect napping spot. I wanted to work part time on my own business, but there was no leftover time or energy between my full-time job and my ongoing sleep deprivation to focus on that goal.

The Life-Changing Moment

In my late thirties, I was searching the internet for a certification program, when I caught a glimpse of a course in sleep sciences. I had no interest in being a sleep sciences coach at the time; I just wanted to take the course to improve my own sleep. I pulled out my credit card, made the purchase, and spent the next three days watching interviews with sleep doctors, reading slides, and making notes. I left the spot on the mattress only to eat and empty my bladder. By the end of the weekend, I had passed the final exam and earned my sleep sciences certification, making me a certified sleep coach.

The most exciting part was not the certification; it was educating myself about sleep. I found the whole thing fascinating. I had learned about all the ways sleep could improve my health and my life, and what happens in our bodies while we sleep. I finally had an appreciation for something I had been purposely avoiding for decades. I was intrigued and wanted to get to work on fixing my sleep as soon as possible, and then I couldn't wait to help others fix theirs.

When I first introduced myself to the online wellness world in summer 2017, I was one of a very small community who focused solely on sleep. Among my business-coaching group of thousands, I was the one and only sleep professional in a sea of personal trainers, dieticians, and weight-loss coaches. Finding clients was easy because I had no competition, and potential clients were asking for help before I felt ready to coach.

Working with women who struggle with insomnia symptoms quickly became my specialty because it hit so close to home. While I was ready to jump into creating multistep evening rituals with clients, they were marveling at the simple, but powerful, truths that I often took for granted. The idea that a client could lie in bed and focus on rest instead of sleep was said to be "life changing." A woman who fought her own negative thoughts night after night felt such freedom after being told her thoughts had no control over her. It was a relief to learn that so many women who suffered from insomnia symptoms and bedtime anxiety didn't need me to give them medical advice (which is a good thing because I'm not a doctor). They needed help relieving stress, dealing with their own negative thought patterns, and perfecting the small sleep habits we often overlook.

I started *The Calm & Cozy Podcast* the following winter and used my platform to share everything I had learned. I told stories about my experiences, offered tips and product reviews, and thrived in a medium that let me use my unique voice to connect with others without ever having to leave the house.

One of the surprising side effects of working with others on improving their sleep is the vast improvements in my own. Paying attention to everyone else's sleep habits has magnified my own habits and practices, and the people in my life are looking to me to be an example.

Every evening when I start yawning, I prepare for bed instead of fighting it. I happily go to bed at a time other people would consider early. I nestle into my bed and smile. I drift off to sleep without a struggle between my brain and the rest of my body. I intentionally wake up before anyone else in my house, and after I get out of bed, I open the curtains, letting the sun stream into my

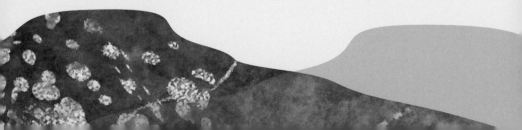

bedroom. I say cheesy things like "What a beautiful morning!" and I spend the first hours of my day moving my body, working on fun projects, and enjoying my time alone. Morning has become my favorite part of every day. Being a night owl no longer serves its purpose, and I realize now that it never really did.

One of the unexpected benefits of improving my sleep is the gift of time. In addition to completing my daily responsibilities, I have more time—I'm talking *hours*—to work out and be the healthiest I've been in decades and to work on my favorite creative projects, including my business, my podcast, my blog, and this book. I can tell you from experience that it's impossible to pursue anything that requires extra time and energy if you're dragging yourself through your day longing for your next nap.

Only You Can Transform Your Sleep Habits

The bad news about transforming your sleep is that no one tip or technique will change everything. I can't give you the one big secret to epic sleep habits—and even if I did, there's no guarantee that one thing would work for you. Different things work for different people, and it's going to take some trial and error to discover what will change how you sleep.

The good news: you most likely have access to everything you need to transform your sleep. You don't need to spend thousands of dollars renovating your bedroom or buying sleep aids. You don't need to change who you are to transform your sleep. What you *do* need to do is make some small shifts in your schedule, your activities, and your mind-set. You also need to be okay with admitting when you could use some help from a professional. Talking to your doctor about your symptoms and going for an overnight sleep study can rule out any underlying issues. It's impossible to get your sleep back on track if you don't know what the problem is.

This book is full of sleep tips and techniques that have the potential to be life changing, but I can't stress enough how important it is that as you work your way through this book, you focus on your thoughts and your words just as much as your actions. You can have the strictest pre-bedtime policies, the prettiest bedroom, and the coziest bed, but if you're clenching your teeth and expecting the worst as you climb into bed every night, you're not doing yourself any favors. Approaching any situation believing it's going to be awful will likely make it awful. Your brain plays just as big a role in your sleep every night as the rest of your body does.

My goal for this book is to change your relationship with sleep and give you a new appreciation for all of the good it can bring into your life. I want you to see getting a good night's sleep as the best way to take care of yourself: the ultimate act of self-care and self-love. I'm also going to arm you with the tools you need to improve your sleep habits, starting today. My wish for you is that by the time you finish reading this book, you will be falling asleep without a struggle and waking up ready to take on the day. I want you to think of sleep as something you *get* to do, not something you *have* to do.

You're going to spend one-third of your life sleeping. Think about that for a moment. How you spend that third will have a significant impact on the health, happiness, and success of the other two-thirds of your precious life, so before we begin, I want to ask you a question:

What life could you be living if you weren't tired all the time?

"*Sleep is the golden chain that ties health and our bodies together.*"

—Thomas Dekker

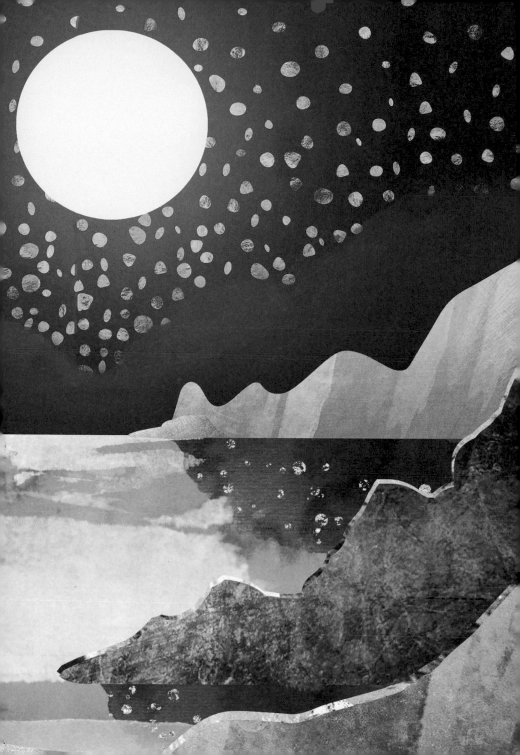

Sleep Basics

WHY SLEEP IS IMPORTANT

From the outside, sleep looks pretty uneventful—lying still, eyes closed, occasional leg twitches—but on the inside, a lot is going on. As you sleep, your body and all of its systems are working hard to repair and replenish. Every system of your body is improved by a good night's sleep. It's like a total body workout for your circulatory, digestive, muscular, nervous, lymphatic, and reproductive systems. Sleep improves your memory, helps reduce stress and anxiety, balances your mood, and boosts creativity. Getting enough sleep can also enhance your immune system during cold and flu season, lower blood pressure, help maintain your weight, lower your risk of diabetes, and keep your heart healthy. Getting your seven to eight hours is excellent for the health of your skin and hair, to maintain their healthy appearance and growth. There is a reason it's called "beauty sleep."

Sleep is the only natural treatment I can think of that can help with almost any problem you may have, even the most difficult challenges you may face. One good night's sleep can make a difference. Sleep restores the body physically, mentally, and emotionally. What's bothering you right now? Sleep can help with that. The positive effects of sleep can be direct, like curing a headache and helping you stay alert during a critical morning meeting, or indirectly, like giving you a break so you can wake up refreshed and ready to strategize and tackle your problems. Sleep doesn't require a prescription or involve a long list of painful or embarrassing side effects. It is the single most helpful tool in your arsenal right now that doesn't cost a penny to use—and that's probably why it's so underrated. Getting a good night's sleep as a way to improve almost anything sounds too good to be true!

THE STAGES OF SLEEP

Research has determined that we experience four stages of sleep, broken into non-REM sleep (stages 1 to 3) and REM sleep (stage 4). REM stands for "rapid eye movement," because during sleep, your eyes move quickly in different directions. The body cycles through each of the four stages—taking approximately ninety minutes—several times per night. Each cycle brings restoration and healing to the body in its own essential and surprising ways:

Stage 1: Light Non-REM Sleep

Stage 1 is a transition and is more the act of falling asleep than a true stage of sleep. The body is in and out of sleep and awakens easily, as we can still hear what's going on around us. The mind drifts off while our brain waves begin to slow and our muscles relax (and often twitch or jerk) as slow eye movement begins.

Stage 2: Light Non-REM Sleep

Stage 2 is a light stage of non-REM sleep that takes up about 50 percent of the night. During this stage, blood pressure and core body temperature drop, breathing slows, and eye movements stop. Light sleep is vital for processing memories and emotions and is known as the general maintenance phase while our metabolism regulates.

Stage 3: Deep Non-REM Sleep

Stage 3 is known as deep non-REM sleep and makes up 12 to 25 percent of our sleep. Our bodies experience more deep sleep during the first half of the night and very little to none during the second half. During this stage, the body is immobile and we do not wake easily. Coincidentally, this is also the phase when sleepwalking and sleep-talking take place. Stage 3 sleep is when most of the body's systems are repaired and replenished. Muscle and tissue repairs happen with the release of a growth hormone and an increase of blood flow and oxygen. Most sleep experts agree that this stage is the most crucial one for the health of the body.

Stage 4: REM (Rapid Eye Movement) Sleep

Stage 4 is called REM sleep and is the most important stage for brain health. This stage happens mostly during the second half of the night. Dreaming and brain activity occur in this stage while the body becomes paralyzed. The breath becomes shallow and irregular, as heart rate and blood pressure rise. Adults spend about 20 percent of their sleep in the REM stage, while infants typically spend 50 percent of the night in this stage.

CALCULATING YOUR BEDTIME

Now that you've learned (or reviewed) the importance of all four stages of sleep, choose a bedtime to make sure you're getting a healthy dose of each stage. From what we've learned about REM sleep, it's a critical stage that happens in the second half of the night, so getting an insufficient amount of sleep means less of the brain-boosting REM stage. Here are the steps for helping you calculate your bedtime:

1. **Aim for five cycles per night.** Aiming for five cycles per night amounts to 7.5 hours of sleep. Here's the math on that:
   90 minutes x 5 cycles = 450 minutes
   450 ÷ 60 (minutes per hour) = 7.5 hours

2. **Decide when you need to wake up.** Choose the time you need to be awake (7 a.m., for example), and then count backward 7.5 hours on the clock. If you don't instantly fall asleep (most of us don't), add 20 to 30 minutes—or however much time you typically need to fall asleep, making your total time in bed roughly 8 hours.

Every hour of sleep accumulated before midnight is worth two after-midnight hours of sleep. Consider it a little bonus, not an added stressor, especially if your work schedule doesn't allow for it. These bonus hours can make your night of sleep feel a little more refreshing.

Going to bed early should benefit you, as long as you are tired at the time. Don't choose a bedtime based on when you think you should go to bed. Choose a time when you typically feel tired. Forcing sleep when you're not sleepy can result in restlessness and insomnia.

If it has been a while since you paid attention to the cues that you are sleepy, try it tonight. When the yawning begins and your eyes start to feel heavy, make note of the time. You don't have to climb into bed after the first yawn, but it's most likely the perfect time to start preparing for sleep.

I was working with a woman who was taking my online course as a beta tester. Let's call her Lee. I was used to my program participants having breakthrough moments during the later modules of the program, but Lee's aha moment came early on, as she calculated her bedtime. Figuring out a time to go to bed based on when she was tired was a new concept to her. Lee had been crawling into bed at a time she believed to be good, even though she didn't have to be up for work until later than most people do. She thought that by spending more than eight hours in bed, she was doing the right thing. It was causing her to spend the early hours of her night lying awake, plagued by restless thoughts and worries. It was a massive relief to Lee to allow herself to go to bed when she was tired, no matter the time, because it meant less worrying and more sleeping.

When you think of the remainder of your evening as a transition into sleep, you become more aware of the decisions you're making and the way they could be negatively affecting your sleep. Is that after-dinner coffee or glass of wine contributing

Do Some People Require Less Sleep?

There is a very small percentage of people on the planet who claim they can function on less sleep than the rest of us. Do they possess a superhuman strength that has yet to be discovered? Studies are currently being done at the University of California on a genetic mutation that allows people to feel fully rested on less than six hours of sleep per night. The study sounds interesting but raises the question, is the idea of less rest a good thing? Does our overworked, overextended, hustle-obsessed society need another excuse to forego stillness and rejuvenation of the mind and body just because we can? If so, meditation and mindfulness practices wouldn't be as wildly popular as they are today. With the rise of minimalism and the constant focus on the decluttering of our homes and minds, many people are linking happiness with seeking less, not more. As a society, we are already chronically busy and stressed, and less time for rest is not the solution.

to your restless hours in bed? Is checking your work email at night adding to your evening anxiety? Would starting a movie earlier give you time to unwind before bed? These are the questions you will start to ask yourself when you think of the evening as a transition into rest.

The hours leading up to your time in bed are going to be the most important in deciding what kind of sleep you're going to have. Ignoring the fact that bedtime is approaching won't make it go away. Give in to the idea that your body craves rest and do what you can to make the hours leading up to that glorious rest as enjoyable and peaceful as possible.

MELATONIN

Melatonin is a hormone made naturally in the body by the brain's pineal gland. Melatonin regulates our sleep-wake cycles—also called our circadian rhythm or internal body clock—and is triggered by our eyes' detection of light and dark. The pineal gland produces melatonin when light is absent in the retina. The pineal gland's peak hours of production are at nighttime, and melatonin is what makes us feel sleepy. When the eye detects a large amount of light during the day, melatonin production drops, causing us to feel awake and maintaining a feeling of alertness throughout the day. In general, the pineal gland turns on in the evening and turns off in the morning, cycling through sleepiness and alertness.

How to Make Melatonin

Let's talk about some of the ways you can work with your body to regulate your sleep-wake cycle and get your body to create melatonin on its own.

Knowing what we do about how light and dark affect our feelings of alertness and sleepiness, think about waking up and creating an environment full of natural light. When your alarm wakes you, turn on a light to signal to your pineal gland that it's time to wake up. Open the curtains, drink your coffee, tea, or smoothie on the front step, and go for a walk if you have time. If you spend time outdoors in the morning, don't put your sunglasses on right away. Leave them off for a few minutes, so your eyes adjust to daylight and your brain gets the signal.

If you work all day in an environment with bright, fluorescent lighting or you stare at a computer screen for hours—or both— take care to spend your evening away from the same light you've been exposed to all day. Blue light can be overstimulating, and your body and brain need some time to relax and unwind before bed. In the evening, dim the lights in your home to prepare your brain for sleep. Use lamps or dimmer switches to keep the lights low and encourage sleepiness.

Avoid screens after sunset. I know that's difficult for a lot of people, myself included, but our constant use of technology is killing our sleep. We have to learn to put down our phones and turn off our TVs and find other things to do in the evening. Replace your screen time with quality family time, or enjoyable alone time. If it's something you look forward to, it will feel less like a consolation.

Taking a hot, relaxing bath can also produce melatonin and make you feel sleepy. Your bath or shower shouldn't happen too close to bedtime because going to bed warm can make it harder to fall asleep. Give yourself an hour between a hot-water soak and crawling into bed.

The body creates a surge of melatonin between 10 p.m. and midnight, so remember that the next time you leave the room to go to bed before everyone else does. As your family members are making fun of you, you can confidently respond, "I have to get ready for bed; I have a hot date with a melatonin surge at 10."

Melatonin-Rich Foods

If you're hungry for an evening snack, try one that's melatonin-rich, like walnuts, pistachios, cherries, goji berries, almonds, pineapple, bananas, or oranges. Foods that are rich in tryptophan can also up your melatonin production. Tryptophan is an essential amino acid and helps produce melatonin. Foods that contain tryptophan and would make a tasty snack are soy nuts, cottage cheese, pumpkin seeds, almonds, and yogurt.

SLEEP AS SELF-CARE

Self-care and hustle culture are both popular. It can be terribly confusing because hustle culture says we need to work hard to reach our goals, no matter the cost. In the same breath, we're told to practice self-care daily, regardless of how busy our lives are.

Can you practice radical self-care every day if you're constantly pushing rest aside to forge ahead with your plans?

My mission in life, and in this book, is to inspire others to see sleep as the ultimate act of self-care and self-love. I do not subscribe to the adage that "sleep is for the weak." I don't believe in putting off rest because "I'll sleep when I'm dead." Sleep is vital for whatever you want in life right now.

Before we dive into how sleep counts as self-care, let's take a deeper look at what self-care is. Self-care is deliberately making your own physical, emotional, and mental health a priority on a daily basis. Self-care is regularly looking out for number one. That doesn't mean you are your only priority, but it means putting yourself at the top of the list.

A myth to dispel is that self-care involves spending large amounts of money on splurges that may put you into debt, ultimately causing anxiety and feelings of hopelessness. Self-care is not a onetime act or once-a-year stay at an expensive spa. It's taking care of yourself while you go about your daily routine, knowing when you need to be nurtured, and making it happen. You can practice self-care daily for free.

Another myth about self-care is that it should make you feel guilty for taking the time to focus on yourself. Self-care is not taking care of yourself instead of taking care of others *(Sorry kids, you're on your own for dinner this weekend—Mommy's practicing self-care!).* It should be done in addition to your other important tasks.

I believe wholeheartedly that the best way to practice self-care is to prioritize sleep. Sleep is responsible for so many healthy mind and body functions. One good night of sleep has a snowball effect, in the same way that one night of poor sleep dictates how the entire next day goes. Diet and exercise get a lot of attention, but one day without exercise or a protein smoothie won't have the same effect that missing a night of sleep will. Diet and exercise have long-term effects on our health, stamina, and mental health, but prioritizing sleep is the easiest way to make it through the day, along with all the long-term benefits that it generates.

Your body is not a machine that works without rest, and you haven't single-handedly discovered the secret to avoiding sleep long term. You need the proper amount of sleep every night, and the people in your life need you to get the proper amount of sleep every night. You have so much to offer the world—how are you going to leave your mark if you're constantly dragging yourself through your day? Get your sleep, friend. The world needs you at your best.

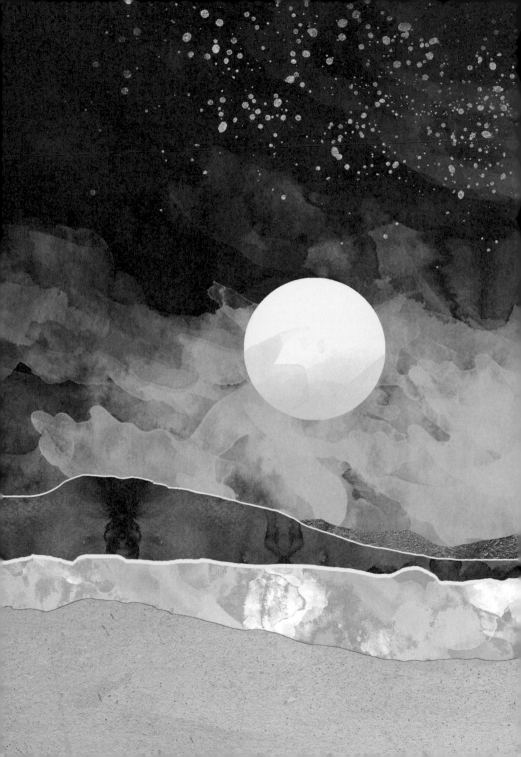

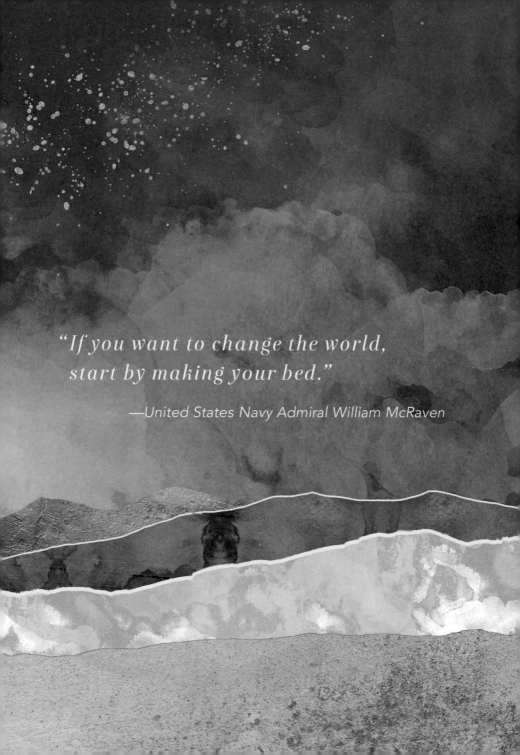

"*If you want to change the world,
start by making your bed.*"

—United States Navy Admiral William McRaven

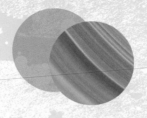

Your Bedroom

PERFECTING YOUR SLEEP ENVIRONMENT

One important aspect of healthy sleep that many people ignore is the state of their sleep space. The overall atmosphere of your bedroom has an effect on the way you sleep, whether you're aware of it or not, and requires attention to the climate, amount of light, color, cleanliness, and design of the room.

Temperature

The temperature of your room should make you want to crawl into your bed and snuggle under the blankets. Our bodies naturally get colder as we're falling asleep and keeping the bedroom cool is consistent with what makes our bodies comfortable. A cooler environment has also been known to stimulate melatonin production (to learn more about this, see page 27), making it easier to fall asleep. You can accomplish this by keeping the temperature between 60 and 68 degrees Fahrenheit (15 and 20 degrees Celsius).

Darkness

For your best sleep, your bedroom should be as dark as possible. Think pitch-black. The simplest way to block exterior light is to invest in a good pair of blackout curtains. Blackout curtains look just like ordinary curtains, but with a heavy fabric that keeps light from passing through.

A pitch-black bedroom also means eliminating all device and appliance lights, no matter how small. If you can, charge your devices in another room overnight or buy blackout stickers to place over the light sources. Digital clocks should be eliminated or turned toward the wall to keep the bright LED digits from glaring at you while you sleep. All visible lights are disrupting melatonin production. Make your bedroom a no-light zone when you go to sleep.

Clutter

Keeping your sleep space free of clutter can be beneficial for your sleep. A messy, crowded bedroom may lead to anxiety and restlessness, making it harder to fall and stay asleep. Try to think of your bedroom as a place of relaxation. It should be an escape from the busyness of the rest of the house.

It is best to keep your bedroom as a space for sleep and sex, and not as a sleep space plus an office or home gym. If possible, keep your bedroom as your bedroom, so it's free from stressors and distractions. If space is an issue and a bedroom office is the only option, try to keep your bed clear of any work and laptops. Your bed should be a place of peace and rest.

Design

An important part of enjoying the time in your bedroom is designing a space that you love. Decorate with colors, fabric, and art that feel good to you. Don't worry about your bedroom matching the rest of the house. Create a space that inspires and relaxes you, and it will be a place you can't wait to retreat to after a long, tiring day.

PICKING A PAINT COLOR

Believe it or not, the color of your bedroom can help or hinder sleep. Bright shades that are beautiful outdoors in nature, like red and golden yellow, can become aggressive on walls. Our brain has an emotional response to color, which is why spas all over the world have used the same shades of muted blue and teal for years.

Your home is a reflection of you and your family, and your bedroom should be a peaceful haven within that space—the place you can go to when the guests have gone and the lights have dimmed. When choosing a bedroom wall color, think of the emotions you want to feel when you walk into the room. If the kitchen and living room are the places you play and laugh and build relationships, the bedroom is the space where you relax, rest, and deepen intimacy with your partner and yourself.

Are the colors in your bedroom supporting peace and rest or are they lively and full of energy?

Paint Colors to Avoid

Bright, loud shades work well in a kid's playroom or a busy family room, but not a bedroom. Paint colors such as red, orange, bright yellow, and lime green can promote feelings of anxiousness and excitement. Avoid dark shades of gray and brown because they can make a room seem gloomy and confining. Bright white can make a space feel sterile and cold, so if you love a white bedroom, opt for an off-white shade.

Paint Colors That Work Well

The many soft, subdued shades of blue, light yellow, and green are great for the bedroom. They alleviate anxiety, promote relaxation, and create a calming atmosphere. If you love color, you don't have to avoid it altogether; look for more delicate hues with gray undertones.

I'll always remember the story of my color-consultant friend who was asked to help choose paint for a client. The paint color was for the kitchen, but later in the conversation she mentioned that her young daughter was having trouble falling asleep and staying asleep. Curious, my friend went into the little girl's bedroom, which had been painted a bright shade of yellow. Fortunately, shortly after her client changed the color to something much softer and lighter, her daughter was sleeping soundly.

ADDING PLANTS

Indoor plants add coziness and warmth to a room while helping purify the air of toxins and pollutants. Certain plants work well in a bedroom because they don't need a great deal of sunlight and care, so don't worry if you don't have a green thumb. The type of

Suggested Bedroom Plants

Aloe vera: Doesn't need a lot of water but loves sunlight; emits oxygen into the air while you sleep; toxic to dogs and cats.

Boston fern: A happy houseplant that likes a lot of light and a daily misting of water; safe for dogs and cats.

Fiddle leaf fig: A suggestion from the "plant guru" in my family as a bedroom plant for intermediate green thumbs. Controls humidity and helps purify the air but is also harder to grow than other plants on this list; must be kept away from air conditioners and heating vents.

Lavender: Has a smell known to improve sleep and increase the amount of deep sleep; should have access to a bright window for a few hours a day; toxic to dogs and cats.

Peace lily: Reduces spores, an excellent benefit for people with allergies; can survive in low to moderate light; toxic to dogs and cats.

Rubber plant: Easy to maintain and keep indoors; prefers moderate to bright light, so place it near a window; toxic to dogs and cats.

Snake plant: Converts carbon dioxide into oxygen and removes toxins from the air; easy to maintain and prefers indirect sunlight; toxic to dogs and cats.

Spider plant: Releases oxygen into the air at night; is low maintenance but hardy; safe for dogs and cats.

plant you choose should depend on the amount of care you can provide in your home. Low-maintenance plants that can thrive without a lot of water and sunlight will do well anywhere, whether you live in a basement apartment or a high-rise condominium with a lot of natural light.

USING ESSENTIAL OILS

Essential oils are aromatic liquids that occur naturally in various parts of plants, herbs, flowers, fruits, woods, and spices. The distilled oils can be used topically as well as aromatically to promote relaxation, relieve anxiety, and calm the nervous system. My favorite way to use essential oils for relaxation and sleep is with an ultrasonic diffuser that disperses vapor into the air. Several essential oils have calming properties you can use alone or in a blend during your evening routine:

Bergamot: calming, uplifting

Cedarwood: calming, soothing, grounding, aphrodisiacal

Clary sage: calming, uplifting, antianxiety, eases emotional tension (avoid during pregnancy)

Cypress: calms the nervous system, relieves insomnia

Frankincense: calming

Geranium: sedating, uplifting, antianxiety

Grapefruit: uplifting

Jasmine: calming, sedating, uplifting

Juniper berry: antianxiety, relieves fatigue and nervous energy

Lavandin: calming, eases insomnia and stress

Lavender: calming, sedating, uplifting, eases insomnia, irritability, and migraines

Lime: refreshing, uplifting

Mandarin/tangerine: sedating, soothing, eases insomnia and nervous tension

Marjoram: sedating, calms the nervous system, eases migraines

Melissa: calming, uplifting (avoid during pregnancy)

Patchouli: calming, uplifting, aphrodisiacal

Petitgrain: calming, uplifting, eases insomnia

Roman chamomile: balancing, calming, sedating

Rose: uplifting, antianxiety

Rosewood: uplifting, antianxiety

Sandalwood: grounding, uplifting

Sweet orange: sedating, uplifting, eases nervous tension

Vetiver: calming, comforting, grounding

Ylang-ylang: calming, balancing, uplifting (use in moderation; may cause headaches)

Lavender

Lavender essential oil is believed to have antiseptic and anti-inflammatory properties, which can help heal minor burns and insect bites. It's useful for alleviating anxiety, insomnia, depression, nervousness, restlessness, migraines and headaches, sleep disruptions, and stomach irritation. Still, lavender is best known for its calming effects.

This aromatic oil blends well with bergamot, grapefruit, mandarin, sweet orange, geranium, frankincense, vetiver, patchouli, cedarwood, and petitgrain oils. Lavender and clary sage oil make the perfect calming blend, as both are sedatives.

Buying Essential Oils

When choosing an essential oil brand, look for "100% pure" and "organic" on the label, with no other ingredients listed on the bottle other than the name of the plant. For example, if you're buying a bottle of lavender essential oil, the label should say "Ingredients: *Lavandula angustifolia* (Lavender) Oil." It will list the botanical name of the oil as well as the more common name. If it contains another oil, such as sunflower oil, for example, the contents have been diluted with a filler oil and are not considered pure.

Essential oils are not regulated, so companies may claim erroneously that their oils are pure and organic. Do your research and look for the highest-quality essential oils you can afford. Before you use essential oils topically, always dilute them in a carrier oil that has little or no scent (such as sweet almond, avocado, or grape-seed oil). Although many essential oils have a gentle and calming scent, they are potent. It takes approximately 3 pounds (1.4 kilograms) of lavender flowers to produce 1 tablespoon (15 milliliters) of lavender essential oil.

When choosing an essential oil, start by smelling the oil in the bottle. Open the cap and hold the bottle several inches from your nose. You'll know right away if it's a scent you like. Oils can have a long list of desirable properties, but if you can't stand the smell, you will never use it.

Diffusing Essential Oils

An ultrasonic diffuser disperses essential oils into the air and is available in a wide range of styles and sizes. Typically, you get what you pay for with diffusers. Note that an ultrasonic diffuser is not the same as a humidifier and that essential oils should not be used in other appliances. A diffuser has a few pieces that fit together, the largest piece being the container that holds the water. Fill with water to the fill line and add drops of pure, undiluted essential oils to the water. Place the lid on the water

Pillow Spray

Another way to use essential oils in your bedroom
is as a pillow spray. High-quality essential oils
are not greasy, so you don't have to worry about
staining your bedding or clothes. Here's a recipe
for a calming spray:

Clean spray bottle
¼ cup (60 ml) water
10 drops lavender essential oil
10 drops chamomile essential oil

Combine all the ingredients in the spray bottle
and shake well before each use. Spray from a few
feet above your pillow or bedding.

container and plug it into the unit. A mist will come out the top
of the diffuser. Place the diffuser in a safe, central location where
it will not be knocked over.

When adding oil to the diffuser, start slowly. Try one drop
and see how you like it. A little goes a long way, and it's better

to gradually add drops than to start over. Before blending oils, remove the caps and hold the bottles close together to smell the blend. It's a less wasteful way to find out if the scents of the oils will work together in the diffuser. When you find a combination you like, write down the names of the oils and the number of drops you added so you can re-create the blend. There's no rule for how many drops of each oil you should use, but some essential oils are more potent than others. Start with one drop of each and add more as you go.

Many essential oil brands create premixed blends, a great way to enjoy the benefits of the oils listed below without having to buy them separately. Here are some recommended blends:

- Bergamot, cypress, and patchouli
- Bergamot, grapefruit, lime, and sandalwood
- Bergamot, grapefruit, orange, patchouli, and ylang-ylang
- Chamomile, lavender, and ylang-ylang
- Lavender, frankincense, and cedarwood
- Lavender, orange, marjoram, and frankincense
- Lavender and vetiver
- Orange, lavender, sandalwood, and ylang-ylang

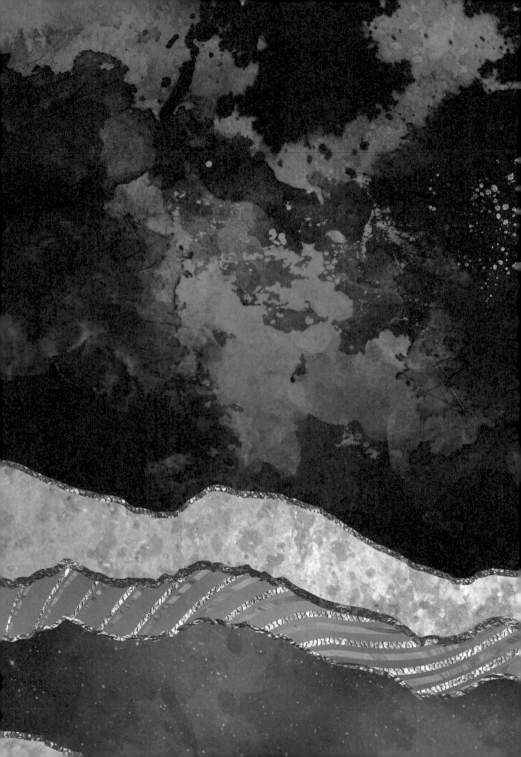

"There is a time for many words, and there is also a time for sleep."

—Homer

Changing Your Thinking about Sleep

CELEBRATING SLEEPINESS

We get tired every night as our bodies prepare for their most difficult and important tasks, and yet many of us still act surprised when our first yawn of the night arrives. It may surprise us that our bodies need sleep and that they start yearning for it around the same time every evening. You are not a wimp for listening to and honoring your body. Stop thinking of going to bed as a sign of weakness. When you think about it, the sleep-wake cycle is a pretty amazing thing. Our natural circadian rhythm, when working correctly, gently nudges us when it is time to rest and wakes us when it is time to start the day. If you begin to feel tired at roughly the same time most evenings and you wake up around the same time every morning, your internal body clock is working. Congratulations! But, if you're fighting these natural feelings of sleepiness, you're competing against nature. Fortunately, it won't take long to get your internal body clock in sync with the rest of your world.

The Sleep Basics chapter (see page 20) discussed the incredible workings of your body and brain during the four stages of sleep. You need to leave room for sleep in your schedule as you would time for meeting up with a friend. Honor your body's way of telling you that it's time to wind down by working with it and not against it. When you start feeling tired in the evening, embrace the feeling and thank your body for doing its job. If you wake just minutes before your alarm rings, take that as a sign that your internal body clock is doing what it should. The best thing you can do at that moment is to get out of bed and start your day. As you do, don't forget to thank your body clock for being so magical.

Choosing Sleep Is a Strength, Not a Weakness

For some reason, we love to make fun of the person who is the first to go to bed. Until I learned to love sleep and appreciate my time in bed as valuable self-care and alone time, I was making those jokes. I used to laugh at the people in my life who went to bed early. I had terrible sleep habits for years, and I used my status as a night owl as an excuse to avoid going to bed for as long as possible. Somehow I thought sleeping less made me cool. Meagan is an early-to-bed person in my life. (She also loves a good nap, like me.) She has been an early riser for years, even as a teenager, and she has always valued a good night's sleep.

Meagan has this thing she does that I've always found hilarious. When we're together in a group and it's later in the evening, at some point she'll get up and leave the room. We would assume that she went to get another glass of red wine or use the washroom. About twenty to thirty minutes later, when it's obvious that she's not coming back, one of the newer people in the group will suddenly notice she's still gone and ask, "Where's Meagan?" One of the regulars who knows her well will answer, "She's in bed. She does that." Can you blame her for sneaking away to go to sleep? If she had announced her departure, someone definitely would have tried to change her mind.

"Well, I'm off to bed. Goodnight, everyone!"

I can hear the groans now. "No! Come on! Stay!" Someone might offer her another drink. Another person might tell her the night is young and so is she.

Why do we do that? Why is going to bed seen as quitting? Fighting our natural urge to go to sleep is not beating nature at its own game. You cannot win this fight. Embrace your body's need to rest as a strength, not a weakness.

The sneak-away-to-go-to-bed move is now one of my favorite party tricks. I'm the one sighing happily in bed upstairs while the partygoers in the family room are trying to hide their yawns or blinking hard to fight off drowsiness.

The next time you're yawning and it's evening, stop fighting it. Your body needs rest, and feeling tired is healthy.

LEARNING TO LOVE SLEEP

Learning to *love* sleep was the single most important thing I did to transform my sleep habits. If you do nothing else, make it your goal to make sleep your friend, no matter how difficult your current relationship with sleep is. Here's why: We naturally avoid doing things we're not good at, and our attitude toward improving the situation is going to be, *I'm not good at this, so why bother?* If you sleep terribly, you probably don't spend a healthy amount of time in bed. Why would you, if your experiences there are mostly negative? If you're approaching sleep as though it's the enemy, you're going to approach it aggressively. This negative attitude toward sleep, no matter how justified, is hurting your chances of achieving happy, healthy sleep habits.

If you're waiting until you sleep perfectly every night to *love* sleep, you're going to be waiting a while. It's time to bury the hatchet. It's time to fake it till you make it and start over with your emotional relationship with sleep—because, let's face it, you can't avoid it forever. The one-third of your life you spend sleeping is passing you by! Here's how you can learn to love sleep:

Change the way you talk about sleep. Stop telling people you slept terribly last night and referring to yourself as a poor sleeper. When you hear yourself speaking negatively about sleep, change the subject. If you have nothing good to say, don't say anything at all.

Stop calling yourself an insomniac if you regularly or occasionally struggle with insomnia. There is nothing positive about that label, and every time you connect yourself with the act of struggling to fall asleep, you make it harder to fall asleep. Come to terms with the fact that sleep doesn't happen instantly to everyone every night and give yourself a break.

Think happy thoughts about sleep. By looking forward to being cozy in your bed with nothing to do but rest, you can flip the switch in your brain and make sleep a new friend rather than a longtime enemy.

My aunt laughed when I told her I was writing a chapter about changing your thoughts about sleep. She waited until I finished rambling and said, "I have a story for you about positive thinking." She went on to tell me about the Egyptian cotton bedding she found when she was shopping one day with her sister. This set of sheets was incredibly soft, but the price tag was too high. She didn't bring them home that afternoon but ended up back at the same store days later. Again she found herself holding the same set of sheets, badly wanting them but resisting because of the price. Nudged lovingly by her shopping companion that day, my aunt finally made the purchase, considering them a treat to herself.

That night, she slid herself into bed and settled in. It took mere seconds to realize she *hated* the new sheets. With the sheets clinging to her legs as she moved, my aunt longed for the familiar feeling of her usual crisp cotton sheets. Sure, her new bedding was soft, but almost too soft. "I hated how they felt against my skin," she said, laughing. "I was so disappointed—and I had already washed them, so returning them wasn't an option."

Don't worry; the story ends happily. You know why? Because my aunt decided she was going to talk herself into loving her new sheets. "Every night, I would get into bed and say, 'Ohh! These sheets are so luxurious! I love how they feel against my skin!'"

Sleep Mantras

If you still need help feeling positive about sleep, create some sleep mantras to help you gradually change the way you speak and think about going to sleep. Here are some suitable (and deliciously cheesy) mantras to try:

I can't wait to go to sleep tonight!
Sleep is going to feel so good. It always does.
I can't wait to get into my cozy bed and go to sleep.

I could picture my aunt giggling to herself as she said it. Believe it or not, her strategy worked. Shortly after buying and hating those Egyptian cotton sheets, my aunt talked herself into loving them.

It's okay if you have to laugh or feel silly while you tell yourself positive things about sleep. You don't have to feel that way now to change how you'll eventually feel. For now, say the words and see how your thoughts start to have a positive effect on the rest of your body.

CHANGING YOUR RELATIONSHIP WITH YOUR BED

How is your relationship with your bed? Do you occasionally struggle with insomnia, restlessness, or waking up for no known reason? I don't blame you if your bed hasn't been your best friend. It's difficult to enjoy spending time in a place that causes stress and negative emotions on a daily basis. Unfortunately, there's no way to avoid going to bed every night. Changing your relationship with it is the simplest and most enjoyable way to take control of the time you're forced to spend there.

Do you love getting into your bed every night? Does your bedding make you want to nestle?

If not, it's time to invest in some bedding you love. Choose fabrics that feel great against your skin, in colors that relax you. Your bed should be amazingly comfortable. You should crawl under the covers every night and let out a happy sigh. When selecting new bedding, ask yourself, *Will this make me happy sigh?* If the answer is yes, it's a winner!

Next, make your bed every morning. Starting your day by making your bed can make you feel as if you've already accomplished something. It's proven to be a habit that can lead to other good habits. A nicely made bed will also make your bedroom appear cleaner and less cluttered.

I agree with the sleep experts who say that the bed is for only two activities: sleep and sex. Your sleep space shouldn't distract

Mattress and Pillow Problems

If your reason for not loving your bed is because you're waking up in pain, you need to take a look at your mattress and pillow. Neck and back pain are common complaints that stem from sleeping on a mattress or pillow that is no longer providing the proper support for your body shape and sleeping positions. When choosing these items, it is best to shop in person, at least at first, so you can try them and know that they're the right size and firmness for you.

you from what it is meant for: rest. This rule works for people struggling with insomnia, and I believe it's also crucial for anyone who is working to repair their relationship with sleep.

Before my sleep improved, I used my bed as my desk while I worked, as a movie-theater seat while I watched movies, and as a craft table. It's no wonder my body didn't know what to do when I finally decided to lie down under the blankets and close my eyes. I was confusing my bed with a place to perform all of my favorite activities.

I will argue that once sleep has become an ally, using your bed for other calming and enjoyable activities turns your bed into a lovely sacred space. Incorporating your bed into your evening routine can be incredibly comforting, not to mention make you feel cozy. When your bed has finally become a calming place of rest, you can undoubtedly enjoy other self-care activities there too. I read in bed, make handmade gifts, and listen to music or podcasts there. These are relaxing activities that can be part of a peaceful evening routine to prepare you for sleep. If you're already in or on your bed when sleepiness hits, you'll have a shorter distance to travel. (After you brush your teeth, of course.)

Your bed has been a place of struggle, unrest, and anxiety for too long. It *should* be your favorite place in the world. When you get into your bed in the evening, I want you to say out loud, "I love my bed." Letting out a happy sigh helps too; I do it every night.

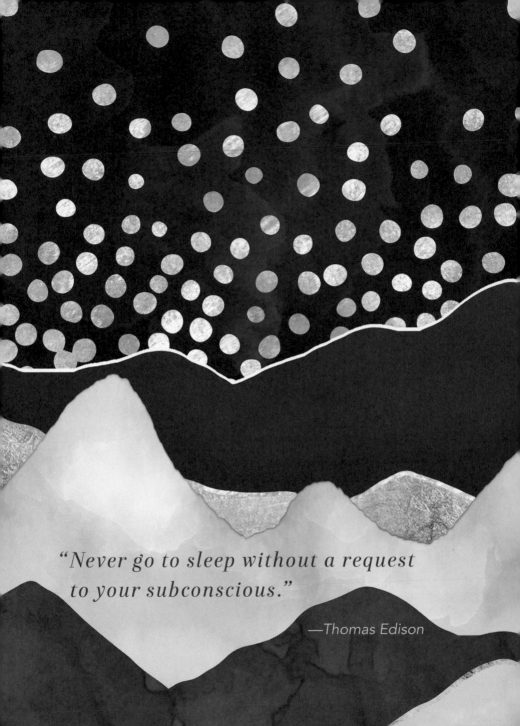

"*Never go to sleep without a request to your subconscious.*"

—Thomas Edison

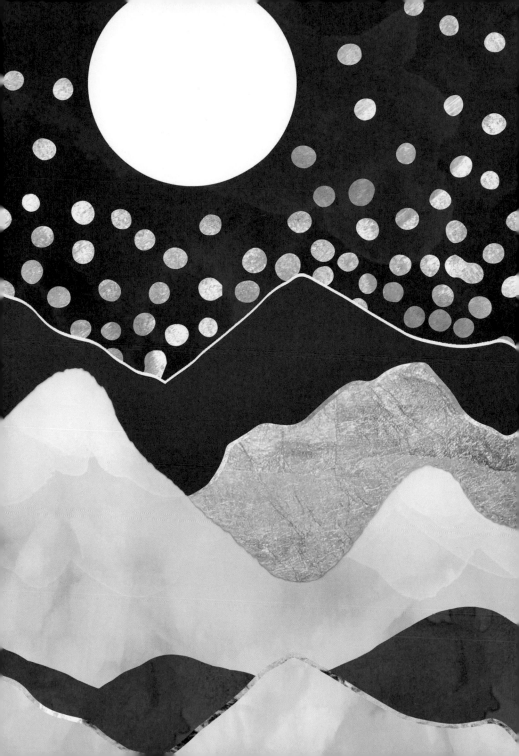

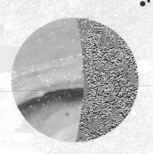

Getting Ready for Bed

TRANSITIONING WITH LIGHT

The easiest way to transition from day to evening is with light. Dimming the lights in a room signals to our brains that it is time to get ready for sleep. When it gets dark, a part of our brains called the pineal gland secretes the hormone melatonin. Melatonin is the hormone that makes us feel sleepy (to learn more about melatonin, see page 27). The blue light emitted from our computers, phones, and television screens blocks melatonin production, tricking our brains and bodies into thinking it is still daytime.

Before the invention of indoor lighting, humans used to go to sleep and wake with the natural cycle of the sun. When it was dark, it was time for bed; when morning came and the sun started to rise, it was time to get out of bed and start the day. Indoor lighting is an incredible invention, but it messes with our bodies' internal body clocks and our sleep-wake cycles. These days we go to bed when we decide to turn off the lights, and we awaken when we choose to turn on the lights. Adopting a regular sleep-wake cycle is the most straightforward step you can take toward getting your sleep back on track.

Tonight, when you start to feel sleepy, practice spending time engaging in activities that relax you and support your transition into sleep. For those of you who are all-or-nothing types, put away all electronic screens forty-five to sixty minutes before bed and adopt a strict tech curfew. If this sounds too hard-core, start by installing a blue light filter on each of the devices you use at night. Some smartphones come with a blue light filter option in the settings, or there are free filter apps you can download. Program the filter to turn off an hour before bed (as a signal to shut off your device) and turn on at the time you usually wake up. The filter will cast a subtle red glow over your screen, protecting your eyes from untimely blue light, allowing your body's natural production of melatonin to continue.

Another way to protect your eyes from blue light is to wear blue-blocker glasses. These glasses are often tinted different colors, like red or yellow, and protect your eyes from specific percentages of blue light, depending on the manufacturer. In the past, blue-blocker glasses were oversize and not at all attractive. Now these glasses are becoming more mainstream with manufacturers offering modern, fashionable styles.

PEACEFUL BEDTIME ACTIVITIES

Now that you have chosen a bedtime, you can design an evening routine to make the transition from day to night even more comfortable. A bedtime routine that engages you in peaceful activities can relieve stress, calm racing thoughts and worries, and prepare your mind and body for rest. Start your routine twenty to thirty minutes before you plan to be in bed. You might find this to be the perfect amount of time to wind down—or eventually you might want more time to yourself. Start small and adjust as you go.

Having a bedtime routine is the adult equivalent of putting on your onesie, brushing your teeth with your Big Bird toothbrush, and crawling into bed to read *Goodnight Moon*. There's a reason children aren't plucked from their current activities and immediately placed in their beds. We would never expect a busy child to instantly fall asleep. They need to have a regular bedtime routine to help them wind down. Why don't we do the same as adults?

The best evening routines should consist of enjoyable, relaxing activities that make you feel calm and sleepy. Here are a handful of activities that have been proven to do just that:

Go for a walk. Walking puts your brain in a meditative state. Being outdoors reduces stress and improves energy levels. Walking also releases endorphins, which reduce stress hormones. All of these things have a positive effect on your sleep.

Listen to calming music. Slow, quiet music can have a relaxing effect on the mind and the rest of the body. It slows the pulse and heart rate, lowering blood pressure and decreasing stress hormones. (Notice I said "slow, quiet music," not death metal or a loud bagpipe solo.)

Read a (real) book. A University of Sussex study done in 2009 found that reading can reduce stress by up to 68 percent. It can immediately transport you into another world and help take your mind off your worries. Reading helps bring on sleepiness, which makes it a tremendous pre-bedtime and bedtime habit.

Work on a creative project. Being creative releases dopamine and endorphins (the happy hormones) and helps relax your mind and body. Activities such as painting, knitting, crocheting, scrapbooking, or playing a calming musical instrument can be soothing to your body.

Meditate and focus on your breathing. Meditation is an excellent way to wind down for the night, let go of the worries of the day, and calm a busy mind. Focusing on your breath, without changing it, can do wonders for people who have a hard time relaxing at bedtime. The point of meditation and breathing exercises is to refocus your attention. It may take some practice to get used to, especially if you have never let go of your thoughts without dwelling on them, but it's a great way to transition into sleep. I go deeper into this topic in the Falling Asleep chapter of this book (see page 74), but for now, here's one of the breathing exercises I do when I'm not able to shut off my brain:

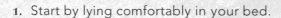

1. Start by lying comfortably in your bed.

2. Close your eyes and take a deep breath in through your nose.

3. Now exhale and picture the air surrounding you as white air.

4. As you inhale through your nose, picture the white air filling your lungs and the rest of your body.

5. On the exhale, picture all the white air leaving your body and filling the space around you.

6. Inhale again through your nose, the white air filling your lungs and your body.

7. And exhale through your mouth, the white air leaving your lungs and your body.

8. Continue to focus on the air filling and emptying your lungs, and when a thought comes into your mind, let it go without reacting to it.

Write in a journal. Journaling is a beautiful way to reduce bedtime worry and stress, increase your time asleep, and improve sleep quality. Stressing or worrying at bedtime can stop your body from winding down, and positive journaling can redirect your thoughts. Here are some different types of journaling to try:

Thought-dumping: With thought-dumping, write down all the things that are bothering or worrying you. Complete the process by closing the book and saying, "DONE!" or something final. If you're writing on a piece of paper, crumple it up and throw it away. The act of getting it all out and then choosing to let go can give you a sense of it being lifted from you. (If you find that dumping those thoughts makes you think about them more and not less, this strategy probably isn't for you.)

Gratitude journaling: Writing about the best part of your day—or ten things you're grateful for right now—has been known to help improve sleep. It's a great practice to help you find the good in your life, especially when things aren't going as planned. It can be as simple as making a list of three to five things or writing, "Today I am grateful for . . . " and letting the words flow.

Letters you don't send: Have you ever been angry at someone, wrote them a message, and then decided not to send it because the act of writing it down was enough? Getting it all out on paper may help you say your piece and move on. The letters can be positive or negative. If someone is on your mind, for whatever reason, take the time to write them a message you don't plan on sending.

New to Journaling?

Here are a few tips to get you started:

1. Choose a journal or notebook that inspires you. For me, it's a book with crisp white pages, no lines, and a beautiful cover that displays a favorite quote. You may already own a journal that fits this description, or you might pick something completely different. Choose a book that makes you want to write in it and grab a pen you enjoy writing with.

2. Get what's in your head down on the page. Don't worry about how it looks or fixing your mistakes or censoring yourself. Just write.

3. End on a positive note. No matter what you're writing about, always end your journaling with a positive note. Look for the lesson in what you just wrote and write it at the end of the page, so you're going to sleep with a pleasant thought as the last thing going through your head.

Tell them how you feel about them and how they have affected your life. Writing directly to that person, even though they won't see it, can bring deep satisfaction and relief. You can decide later whether it's a conversation worth having in real life—or even a letter to send!

Future plans: Use your journal to dream. Write down your bucket list, all the places you would like to go, or the things you want to pursue in the year ahead.

To-do lists: If your brain will not turn off at night because you have a lot to do the next day, making a to-do list can be incredibly helpful. Write down everything that needs to be done, and then place the list where you will see it in the morning. When your list is finished, say out loud, "Tomorrow is taken care of," and go to bed. You can add the list to your phone in the morning if that's how you keep track of tasks you want to accomplish.

Do not take a hot bath or shower. Hot water from a bath or shower raises your core body temperature— and jumping into bed while still warm gives your body the additional task of cooling down. Sleep thrives in cooler temperatures and going to bed warm and sweaty can result in restlessness. If you enjoy a hot bath or shower in the evening, give yourself forty-five minutes to an hour to cool down before climbing into bed.

Do not drink liquids (especially caffeine and alcohol). The first problem with drinking any liquid, even water, too close to bedtime is that it may disrupt your sleep by requiring several trips to the bathroom. The second problem is that half of the caffeine from a coffee, tea, or energy drink stays in your system for several hours. The caffeine can keep you buzzing long after your usual bedtime. Alcohol disturbs REM sleep, which is the most rejuvenating sleep phase. It takes about one hour for your body to metabolize a standard-size alcoholic drink, so you can still enjoy your favorite cocktail with dinner if you're leaving enough time before going to bed. As a rule, cease all liquid consumption at least one hour before bedtime.

Do not vigorously exercise. Exercise is great for improving your sleep, but an intense and sweaty workout too close to bedtime can make it difficult to fall asleep. End your intense workout at least an hour before bedtime, for the same reasons you shouldn't take a hot shower before jumping into bed. Stick to relaxing movement in the evening, such as stretching, walking, or yoga.

BEDTIME RITUALS FOR BUSY PEOPLE

So what do you do if you don't have thirty minutes to relax before bed? I believe it is possible to create a peaceful evening ritual that prepares you for a restful sleep. You don't even have to clear the extra time for it in your already hectic schedule.

How? Let me ask you a question. What do you do before you get into bed? What are the three things you do every night, without fail, no matter how busy your day was? Most people would say they brush their teeth, wash their face, and change their clothes. Maybe you choose your outfit for tomorrow. Think back to when you were a kid getting ready for bed. What did that look like for you?

For most of us, it probably looked something like this. Right in the middle of whatever you were having fun doing, an adult announced that it was time to get ready for bed. You brushed your teeth and emptied your bladder. You changed into your pajamas. You climbed into bed and spent time reading your favorite storybook or looking at the pictures while an adult read to you. Maybe they also sang you a song. When your eyes couldn't stay open any longer, the lights would go out, and you were left to fall asleep in your bed, tucked in beside your stuffed animals.

Now try to re-create this routine, minus the butt-flap jammies. It worked for us when we were kids, so why wouldn't it would work as adults? Here's what you need to do:

1. **Dim the lights.** Turn off overhead lights and use lamps or lights with dimmer switches. Make it sleepy.

2. **Choose your peaceful background sound(s).** Play calming music, or listen to a podcast while you go about your ritual. Too busy to read a book? This is the perfect time to listen to the audio version.

3. **Perform your pre-bedtime wash-up routine.** But don't rush through it—be methodical. Pat your face dry and apply whatever skin products you wear to bed. Give yourself a mini face massage while you're at it. You've had a long day. See what we're doing here? We are turning the mundane task of getting ready for bed into a nightly spa-like ritual. And believe it or not, repeating an activity the same way before bed every night can signal to your brain that it's time for rest.

Whatever you do every night to prepare yourself for bed can be a peaceful bedtime routine. It doesn't have to be mind-blowing or game changing. Use what you're already doing instead of adding more activities to your already busy schedule. If these are the things you do before bed every night, craft them into a slow and simple routine. Do them in roughly the same order every night to signal to your brain that it's bedtime.

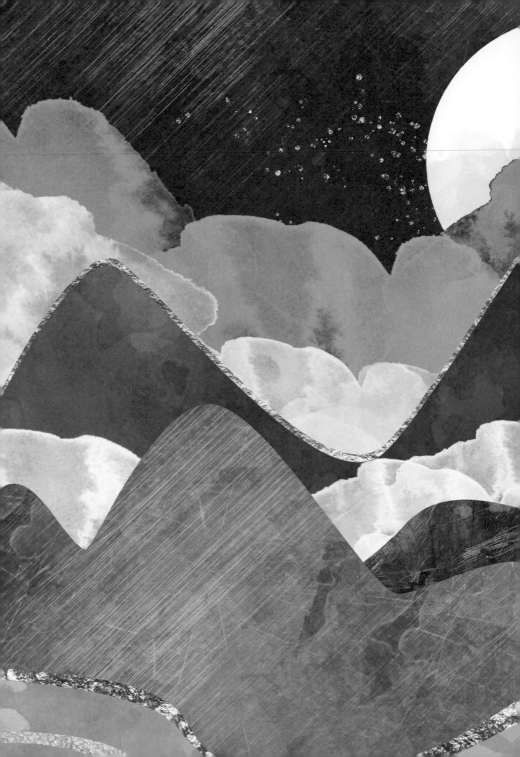

"*Never waste any time you can spend sleeping.*"

—Frank H. Knight

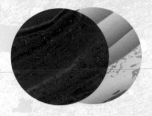

Falling Asleep

SLEEPING POSITIONS

Most people believe they are doomed (or blessed) to sleep in one position for the rest of their lives. Our bodies typically prefer the position they have chosen since childhood (and for some since the womb), but that doesn't mean you can't make changes as an adult.

I was a side sleeper for decades. My body liked that position, with a fluffy down-filled pillow, so I'm sure you can appreciate my disappointment when much of my sleep training told me sleeping on my back was the ideal position. With time and practice, I came to like sleeping on my back, finding myself waking up less because there was no reason to flip over. My back-sleeping skills were already perfectly timed with recovery from surgery that had me propped up on pillows for weeks. I slept well during that time because I was already an award-winning back sleeper.

After an appointment at an overnight sleep clinic, a few years after switching to sleeping on my back, I was diagnosed with very mild sleep apnea that happened only when I slept on my back. I was told to sleep on my side (a suggestion that made me laugh), so I switched back. I tell you this thrilling but heartbreaking tale to say that sleeping positions aren't life sentences and encourage you to make a change if your current position isn't working for you.

On Your Back

Some research has found that sleeping on your back is the best sleeping position for most people. It can prevent neck and back pain while maintaining a neutral position for your neck and spine. It reduces acid reflux because your head is elevated above your stomach. Not having your head crammed into a pillow can help minimize wrinkles. Sleeping on your back is not ideal for people who snore or suffer from sleep apnea because it blocks your airway.

On Your Side

Sleeping on your side is considered a pretty good position. It's suitable for snorers and people with sleep apnea because your airway stays clear. Sleeping on your side is best if you are pregnant and past your first trimester, as it's ideal for blood flow to the uterus without applying pressure to the liver. The left side is preferred, but the right side is also safe for the baby, if it's more comfortable.

In the Fetal Position

Sleeping in the fetal position is considered a not-so-great position. It can increase arthritic pain, because your knees are bent for hours and your neck and spine are curved. But it is a suitable position if you snore, because your tongue isn't restricting your breathing.

On Your Stomach

Considered the worst sleeping position, sleeping on your stomach is bad for your back, putting strain and pressure on your spine. To breathe, you have to turn your head to the side, a position that twists your neck and spine. On a positive note, stomach sleepers can find relief from snoring and sleep apnea.

The bottom line on sleeping positions, according to a sleep coach? (Ahem. Me.) I believe that the best position is the one most comfortable for you. If you can spend the night in that position and wake up with no pain, and if it brings you comfort in other ways, you have found the perfect sleeping position.

PETS ON THE BED

This is a controversial topic, and you probably won't like me very much after this chapter, but it needs to be said. If your cat or dog sleeps on your bed at night and it is disrupting your sleep, it's time to reevaluate your sleeping situation.

I get it. We love our pets, and it feels impossible to say no when they jump up on the bed and start to settle in for the night. It's a comfort to have a creature who loves you unconditionally curled against the small of your back, and how cute does Charlie look with his little head on your partner's pillow? I know firsthand how sweet it is—until it all goes wrong. Your pet starts twitching, twirling, and hogging the duvet, preventing you from flipping over. A few hours later, the resentment arrives and come morning, you're blaming your beloved furry friend for your restless sleep. Then as if to rub it in, while you're yawning uncontrollably and grinding pounds of coffee beans, Buster curls into a ball on the cold kitchen tile, right in front of you, for the first of thirty naps for the day.

Must be nice, fur face.

From the outside, the solution is pretty simple. If your friend was complaining about her terrible sleep and it all stemmed from allowing an animal to sleep on her bed, and she asked you for advice, you would tell her to stop allowing the animal on the bed. But most of us won't take our own advice, especially when we're staring into those sad, puppy-dog eyes.

You are not a horrible pet owner by valuing your sleep more than your dog or cat's temporary desire to cuddle. Your pet doesn't have to be anywhere the next day and will likely spend the next several dozen hours sleeping. Your pet has no responsibilities tomorrow besides looking adorable and chasing squeak toys. I also want to remind you that dogs and cats often choose to sleep on wood and tile floors, not to mention weird places cats inhabit, like empty bathtubs or on top of the refrigerator. It is not cruel to keep your pet off your bed at night so that you can get a good night's sleep. That's what pet beds are for. Some pet beds are even more comfortable than human beds. Believe me, I've tried them.

It will take superhuman strength to avoid eye contact with your adorable four-legged family member as you close the bedroom door, leaving them in the hall. You will feel like a terrible human being, but I promise you, the greeting you get the next morning when your pet sees their favorite person emerge well rested and ready to play fetch will be worth it.

So as you enforce a "humans only" bed rule, repeat this to yourself when the guilt starts to set in: "My sleep is essential, and [name of pet] will be fine." And then keep saying it until you believe it.

If you allow your pet to sleep on the bed because it's easier than dealing with the noise they'll make if they're kicked out, that's another issue you'll have to resolve. Is there a room far enough away from yours that will contain their sounds of disapproval? Would wearing earplugs, or using a white noise machine (or app) drown out the paw scratches on the other side of the door? If all else fails, you might have to decide between the lesser of two evils: your sleep with Buster on the bed or your sleep with Buster crying in the hall.

HAPPY COUPLES WHO SLEEP IN SEPARATE BEDS

Perhaps even more controversial than the topic of pets on the bed is the discussion of couples sleeping separately. I'm here to tell you that it's possible for two people who love each other to make incompatible bed partners. I'm also here to assure you that your happiness together does not depend solely on the distance between your bodies as you sleep.

"I can't settle until my husband is beside me," one friend admitted. "I can't sleep alone anymore. I need my wife beside me in bed," another one told me.

That's all very sweet, but what about the rest of us? The couples who dearly love each other but for some reason don't sleep well together? For many happy partners, sharing a bed means waking up exhausted and resentful, but the idea of sleeping apart has never been an option they considered.

My parents were one of those couples.

My mom and dad have been married for more than forty years and shared a double bed for most of them. My mom was always cold at night and needed to warm her feet on my dad's legs. My dad was a kicker, often stabbing my mom with a sudden knee jerk in the middle of the night. They were happy together during their waking hours but weren't finding the nights exactly magical. Whenever my mom would suggest that they sleep separately, my dad would discourage it.

"Your dad didn't want to sleep apart," Mom told me. "He didn't think it would be right."

To me, this logic is funny. (No offense, Dad.) Maybe it's because I've slept alone most of my life, despite having been in happy relationships along the way, but I don't see the connection between loving my spouse and sharing a mattress with him while we're asleep.

It wasn't until my mom had knee-replacement surgery that she started sleeping apart from my dad. My dad, the kicker, didn't want to accidentally hurt her already sore knees, so he slept in the guest room during her recovery. Soon after, my parents started to enjoy the perks of having separate beds. My mom could bundle up under several blankets to stay warm while my dad could spread out. He also didn't have to worry about sneaking in quietly, in fear of waking her up if he stayed up past her bedtime.

"We enjoy having separate beds, and we're still happily married," my mom said recently. "We might even be happier because we're so well rested." Well, it only took forty years!

What about Sex?

Some common reasons for wanting to sleep apart might be that your partner snores. Or you snore and you feel terrible that you're the only one getting restful sleep. Perhaps one of you is a light sleeper and senses every movement the other makes. Maybe your bed is too small or one of you is a blanket hog. Whatever the reason or reasons, stop letting it affect your sleep and embrace the solution.

Do you want to know what's terrible for a relationship? Sleep deprivation. Waking up resenting the person you love for something they have no control over. Isn't it better to move to the couch or the guestroom—or get another bed?

Okay, go ahead. I know you're dying to ask the question I get most while discussing the option of sleeping separately.

Won't sleeping in separate beds hurt our sex life?

My response: Would you be willing to walk across the hall or into the next room to be intimate with the person you love? If the answer is yes, then I'm not worried about your relationship, and you shouldn't be either. A couple with a healthy sex life is probably not into it purely because it's convenient to have their partner beside them every night.

One great idea would be to have sex before departing for your separate rooms. It takes only a few moments to stand up and walk away. This is not a long-distance relationship, honey, it's just a second bed. You'll be fine.

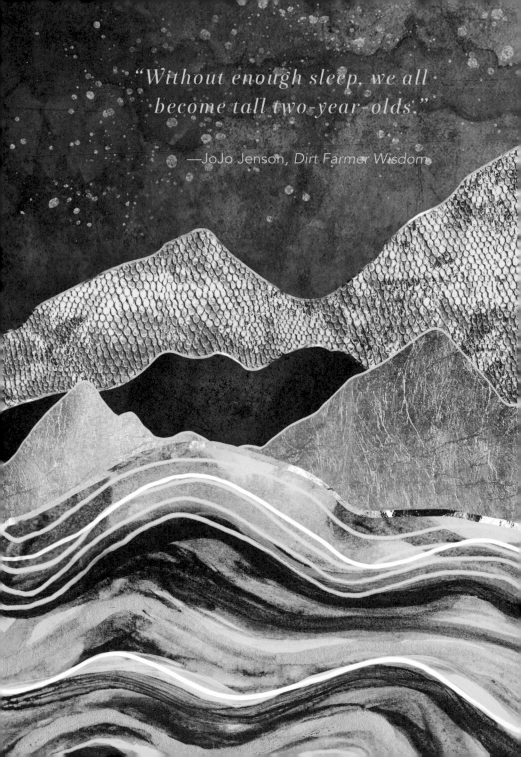

"*Without enough sleep, we all become tall two-year-olds.*"

—JoJo Jenson, *Dirt Farmer Wisdom*

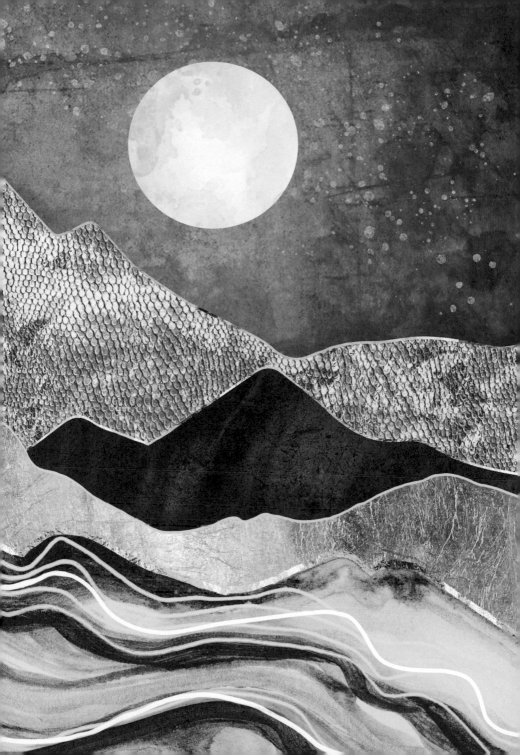

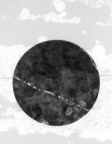

Using Sleep Aids

WHITE NOISE

If you're a light sleeper who wakes up often due to noises inside the house or outside on the street, let me introduce you to my old friend—and perhaps your new best friend: white noise.

White noise works by drowning out the sounds that commonly wake us or keep us from falling asleep. It's produced by combining sounds of all different frequencies. It sounds like static and can vary in tone and volume. As a steady sound that is also predictable, white noise holds your attention without requiring focus.

A few of the sounds in nature that count as white noise are rain, waterfalls, wind, and crashing waves. White-noise machines and apps often include nature sounds, which is good news if you love the sounds of being outdoors without having to go camping or sleep in the backyard.

White-noise machines allow you to select the frequency, volume, and length of the sound you find relaxing. Some people prefer to listen to white noise while they're falling asleep—for the first hour or a few hours—and some keep it on all night. White-noise smartphone apps are good, too, and many are free to download, but may offer fewer options or require you to keep your phone on and running the entire night. An oscillating fan is also a version of white noise, so you may already have something in your home that you can use.

If you want to try white noise to help you fall asleep and stay asleep, it's best to use a constant sound. As much as you may love the sound of a thunderstorm, the sudden crashing bouts of thunder can repeatedly wake you up. The same goes for any noise that sporadically changes in volume, like voices during conversation. Sudden noises can disrupt your sleep and prevent you from getting into your deeper sleep phases, and that will make your sleep restless and unrefreshing.

EARPLUGS AND SLEEP MASKS

If you are a light sleeper who is often awakened by sounds and light streaming into your bedroom, the use of a simple sleep aid or two can make a world of difference. Do what you can to make your sleep space as dark and quiet as possible, but some nights, these things will be beyond your control.

Earplugs

Wearing earplugs can help you sleep through many quieter sounds, like a toilet flushing or roommates chatting downstairs, but still allow you to hear loud, high-pitched noises like the ringing of a phone or smoke alarm.

Earplugs are typically made of foam, which makes them inexpensive. If you are repeatedly waking up in the morning with earplugs lost in your bedsheets, they're too small for your ears. Try a larger size or a different shape. If you're waking up in the middle of the night with your ears aching, the earplugs are too large.

Sleep earplugs are a popular item for people who can't find a foam pair that fits. You're going to pay more, but you'll get a higher quality pair made especially for wearing comfortably at night. If you use earplugs regularly, it can be worth it to pay more for a pair that fits you perfectly, stays in your ears until morning, and lasts a lot longer than a disposable pair.

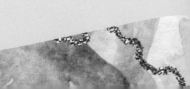

I find that earplugs double as tiny white-noise machines, since they amplify the sound of my breathing, helping me relax.

Sleep Masks

Sleep masks come in different sizes, styles, and designs. They typically take some time getting used to because they cover your eyes and stay on your head with a stretchy elastic band. A good sleep mask will block out all light, something that is particularly helpful for people who sleep beside someone who watches television, works on a laptop, or uses a lamp to read.

If your bedroom is bright in the morning and you're not quite ready to get up with the rising sun, you will probably find a sleep mask helpful—a godsend, even. Like earplugs, sleep-mask designs are improving and evolving. If you shop around and spend a little more, you can find a mask made of comfortable, breathable fabric with a custom adjustable fit.

SYNTHETIC MELATONIN

In pill form, melatonin can be a bit controversial because it comes with its own set of side effects, warnings, and possible interactions. It certainly doesn't help that it's available among the over-the-counter products in the health food section of grocery stores.

Melatonin has side effects that include headache, feelings of depression, daytime sleepiness, dizziness, stomach cramps, and irritability. I asked a handful of my online friends about their side effects from melatonin. Their responses included suffering from scary and disturbing nightmares, waking up feeling hungover and groggy, becoming dependent on it to fall asleep every night, and feeling "totally destroyed" in the morning. The literature about melatonin warns of possible drug interactions with sedatives, birth control pills, and caffeine.

If you're suddenly having problems sleeping and you automatically reach for synthetic melatonin, you're self-diagnosing and self-prescribing without knowing what the real issue is. Before taking melatonin pills, I suggest talking to a qualified professional, as melatonin is not an herbal supplement you should run to every time you have a rough night's sleep.

Could your sleep issue be a symptom of another problem? Could it be eased by managing stress, going to bed at a different time, or spending your hour before bed preparing for sleep instead of cramming in one more episode of a television series?

And if your sleep issues continue, you should see your doctor and ask about a sleep study to rule out other causes.

EXERCISE

I included exercise in this chapter for a reason. You know those days when you spend hours doing something labor-intensive—like helping a friend move, painting the house, or walking around Disney World for twelve hours—and then say out loud, "Wow, I am going to sleep well tonight!"? You predicted that an active day was going to help you sleep. You were right.

Exercising regularly, even for ten minutes a day, can help you fall asleep faster, improve sleep quality, increase the length of your sleep, reduce stress and anxiety, and relieve insomnia. Exercise can improve the body's natural sleep-wake cycle by promoting daytime alertness and helping you feel sleepier at night. If you want one more reason to work out regularly, physical activity increases the time spent in deep sleep, which is the most restorative phase. It also lowers your body temperature as you're cooling down from your workout, and this puts your body in a more relaxed state for falling asleep. Just five minutes of exercise can initiate antianxiety reactions in the body.

Just be careful not to go to bed too soon after a big, sweaty workout. Your elevated hormone levels and core body temperature can make it harder to fall asleep. Leave at least an hour after finishing a tough exercise before climbing into bed.

A Case for Morning Exercise

I am a fan of morning workouts—and that's ironic because I'm not a morning person. I hate getting out of bed, but looking forward to my workout makes it easier to drag myself out from under the covers. I also find the sunshine and fresh air help wake me up, even if it's just a short walk to my car to drive to the gym.

Cortisol levels peak in the morning, causing the body to feel awake and alert. Cortisol is the hormone responsible for regulating mood, providing an increase in motivation, and is best known for the "fight or flight" response. A morning workout will help you take advantage of your body's natural energy boost around that time. Exercise gives you more energy during the day, and when cortisol levels dip in the evening, you can start transitioning into your peaceful pre-bedtime routine.

Starting the day by moving your body will help tire you out later, and the exposure to light first thing in the morning can help increase melatonin levels as bedtime approaches. Our bodies are amazing and perfectly primed for helping us start the day with energy and ending our day peacefully. Working with your body's internal body clock will have a positive effect not only on your sleep at night, but also on every system of the body.

NAPPING

I come from a long line of champion nappers. Both of my grandmothers could fall asleep sitting up while watching a noisy game show. My mom and her siblings can nap pretty much anywhere if they can find a suitable object to use as a pillow. My dad and his brother can put on their football jerseys, make snacks, and settle in to watch a Sunday afternoon game, only to be snoring shortly after kickoff. Napping is in my genes, and I admit that an afternoon nap is one of my favorite things in the world.

My friends often see me leaving an afternoon event to find a nearby place to sleep. If I feel the need to nap, it doesn't matter where I am or who I'm with: if there's an opportunity to sneak away to find a soft spot, I'll do my best to make it happen.

Napping is a perfect way to restore energy, boost creativity, sharpen mental focus, eliminate headaches and fogginess, and take a break from a mentally stimulating or physically demanding activity. A good number of sleep experts think naps are detrimental to our sleep at night and discourage napping at all costs. Other experts praise napping as a great way to recharge our batteries in the middle of a busy day. My opinion is that if you feel the need to sleep during the day, and are able to, controlled naps are amazing when paired with healthy, nightly sleep habits.

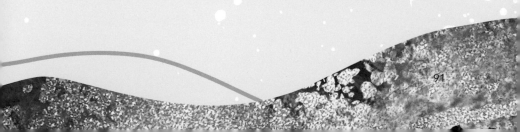

Our bodies experience a natural dip in energy during the early afternoon. (I call it "hitting a wall." That's a metaphor, of course. Be careful out there.) Needing a short nap sometime between lunch and near the end of the workday is normal and does not necessarily mean you are sleep-deprived. Or lazy. I'll go into this more in the Waking Up chapter, but your chronotype (see page 115) will give you more insight into the times of day you feel most awake and most tired, as it refers to your specific sleep patterns. The four chronotypes (bears, wolves, lions, and dolphins) came into the mainstream in Michael Breus' 2016 book, *The Power of When.* It can be a relief to some people to discover their need to nap in the afternoon is something they were born with, and has nothing to do with how they slept the night before.

I believe you should sleep when you're tired, though I have four rules:

Choose the right time of day. As a general rule, you should be waking up from your nap at least four hours before you go to bed for the night. If you're waking up just in time to get ready for bed, you will likely have a problem. People who claim they can't nap because it hurts their sleep later should experiment with napping earlier in the day. It might be that they're taking a break too close to bedtime.

Set an alarm. Timing your nap will help ensure that your sleep is refreshing. Not setting the alarm can result in oversleeping, experiencing grogginess, sleeping through scheduled events, and for some people, uncomfortable hallucinations upon waking. If you nap long enough to enter into the deep sleep stages, about thirty to forty-five minutes after falling asleep, you will wake up feeling tired and disoriented. Waking up in the middle of a deep sleep, especially REM sleep, makes for a nap that is more tiring than refreshing. If you're looking for an energy boost, sleep for ten to twenty minutes. If you need a memory boost, go for an hour-long nap. Sleeping for ninety minutes will complete a sleep cycle, which can be helpful if you need to tackle a big project or test.

Make it cozy. I could also call this third point "Just because you *can* doesn't mean you *should*." If you're tired and have committed to taking a nap, get comfortable. You might have a gift for falling asleep anywhere, but that doesn't mean it's going to be productive, refreshing sleep. Your bobbing head or slowly gaping mouth is going to be disruptive. Find a place to lie down. Turn off the lights and find a blanket, if you can. Make that nap count!

Stop worrying about what other people think. Too many people care about how it looks to other people when they need to lie down. Let them make fun of you for sleeping when you're tired. People who don't appreciate a good nap will likely never understand, and frankly, they're missing out. Don't let someone else talk you out of taking a well-deserved break when you need one.

In my late twenties, I lived for three months in Brasov, Romania. I was volunteering there and was fortunate enough to stay in a house with four other volunteers who were women my age. I would get up early and spend the morning at the hospital where I was working as a muralist. During my walk home I would often take the long way, stopping to see the sights and taking photos. When I finally arrived home a few hours later, I would take a nap in my room, away from my roommates. The women I lived with, although we all got along famously, thought it was strange that I napped daily. For me, it had been a long, exciting day, and ending it with a short nap gave me relief and some time alone.

I had been in Romania for several weeks when one of the other girls showed up in my room with an announcement: "I was feeling tired earlier, so I thought I would pull a Beth and have a nap. I feel amazing! I can't believe I've never thought of this before!" We laughed about it, and for the duration of my time living there, she would often disappear to enjoy a short, refreshing nap.

The "Coffee Nap"

There is also such a thing as a "coffee nap."
This might be just the thing you "I can't nap" people have
been waiting for. It involves drinking a cup of coffee, then
taking a ten- to twenty-minute nap. Caffeine takes about
twenty-five minutes to fully absorb into your bloodstream. By
the time you wake up, you will be alert and ready for action.

It doesn't occur to some people that a nap is an option when they're feeling tired. They clearly didn't grow up as I did, in a household with group nap times on a quiet Sunday.

Some people are convinced that sleeping during the day makes them feel more tired or makes it harder for them to sleep at night. If you need a nap and you have an opportunity to take one, do it. If you're afraid you'll feel worse after waking up, experiment with the time of day and the duration of your naps and set an alarm to prevent oversleeping.

If you've tried everything and you're still not a napper, that's okay. Just rest your body instead. But do me a favor and support the nappers in your life. They're not lazy. They need to lie down every once in a while—or even every day.

I will probably always have people in my life who think my love for naps is amusing, and that's fine. I'll be over here, exhaling loudly under my favorite blanket.

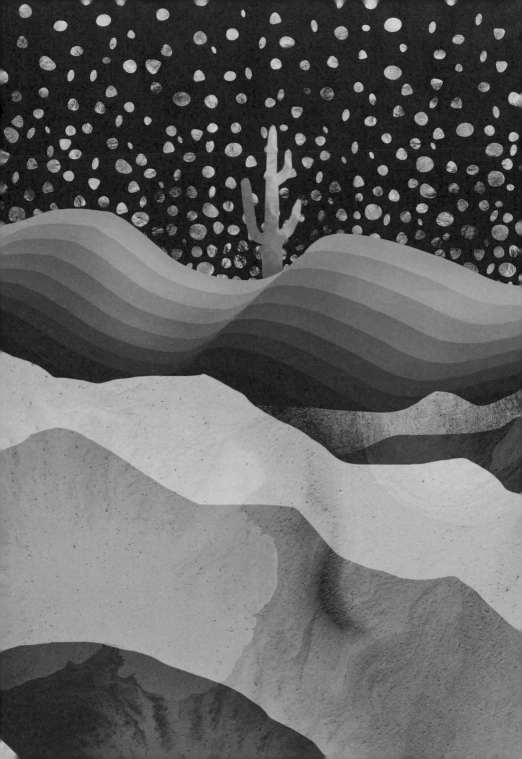

"A ruffled mind makes a restless pillow."

—Charlotte Brontë

While You're (Supposed to Be) Sleeping

FOCUSING ON REST

You're not going to sleep perfectly every night. Occasionally, you will wake up in the middle of the night for no reason, and you're not always going to fall back to sleep quickly and peacefully. A "normal" sleeper understands this and doesn't get stressed out when they have a rough night now and then. But a person who struggles with insomnia, bedtime anxiety, and racing thoughts will find this kind of night frustrating and disappointing. Instead of thinking it's a minor setback, they may think they are to blame. If the night wasn't a good one, they must have done something wrong.

Why does this keep happening? What's wrong with me?

My best advice is to be still and rest. Don't flip over fifty times, hit your pillow, or scream into your duvet. None of those things are restful. This advice is incredibly simple but has been life changing for many who put it into practice. When you're having one of those nights, repeat this to yourself: "Tonight I am resting. My body loves to rest."

I was first inspired by the idea of focusing on rest by my partner, Jake. When Jake was a child and couldn't fall asleep, his mother would tell him to stop worrying about falling asleep and rest instead. Dr. Nerina Ramlakhan's book *Fast Asleep, Wide Awake* confirmed my mother-in-law's genius advice with her own mantra: "If I can't fall asleep tonight, I will rest." I have been obsessed with rest ever since.

Yes, your body also needs sleep, but don't underestimate the value that rest has on your body and your mind. The options are not to sleep or be tortured, and the pressure you're putting on yourself doesn't help, especially when you're already anxious about the situation. You need to change the way you think about your moments awake in bed.

In the past, when you were lying in bed, unable to fall asleep, you were awake. From now on, when you're in bed, I want you to replace "awake" with "resting" as the only other option. If you're not sleeping, you're resting. Embrace rest as the antidote to not being able to sleep—and find peace in the fact that rest is good for you too.

Should You Get Out of Bed?

This is an excellent time to talk about getting out of bed when you can't sleep. If you're going to bed and lying there awake for quite a while, perhaps you're going to bed too early. It should take you about ten to fifteen minutes to fall asleep. If it's taking longer, try moving your bedtime a half hour later.

You should be going to bed feeling tired, but the goal is to be tired, not exhausted. Falling asleep within seconds of your head hitting the pillow sounds like an incredible skill to have, especially if you can fall asleep anywhere, but it could be a sign of sleep deprivation (unless that's typical for you). If it takes you fewer than ten to fifteen minutes to fall asleep, you might want to try going to bed earlier.

If you're regularly having problems falling asleep at night or falling back to sleep after an unexpected wake-up in the middle of the night, I don't suggest getting out of bed to do something else. Sleep experts have differing opinions on this and I am probably going to start a debate, so hear me out before you swear under your breath and close the book. I have a few reasons for believing it's best to stay in bed if you can't fall asleep.

By leaving your bed, you're telling yourself that sleep is the only goal of being there. You're training your body and your brain to put all of your focus on sleep and to retreat if it doesn't work right away. You are placing the expectation on yourself to fall asleep by a specific time, a mind-set that will most likely result in more anxiety. I want you to be comfortable with resting. I want you to spend time in bed without watching the clock or being hyperaware of how much time is passing.

If your reasons for getting up and doing something else are to make you feel tired, then you either weren't tired enough the first time or your body and brain need to unwind first. The solutions are to move your bedtime later, so you feel tired enough to fall asleep, or to use a self-soothing technique to relax your mind.

Another reason I don't want you to leave your bed is that only a tiny handful of activities won't push sleep even further away than it already is. No doubt your home has many screens you can use to distract yourself and pass the time. Reaching for a bright, glowing, melatonin-blocking screen will hurt your chances of falling back to sleep. The news is full of upsetting stories and social media can get us riled up and emotional within seconds. Going for a little walk around the house can raise your stress levels if you notice a mess left in the living room or dirty dishes in the sink. It's also possible that a family member or pet could hear you awake in the house and come to join you, adding to your list of loved ones you now have to tuck into bed for a second time, including yourself.

As someone who has struggled with racing thoughts at bedtime, I know that it only takes a moment of distraction to get your thoughts into a downward spiral, and by staying in bed and choosing to rest, you are eliminating those possible distractions. Rest is the beautiful in-between you can turn to when sleep isn't happening—and unlike sleep, it's always there when you need it.

DEEP BREATHING AND MEDITATION

Deep breathing techniques and meditation can help calm restless thoughts by focusing your thoughts on your breath and your body. Both practices can help you connect to your body, diverting busy thoughts and worries, and signaling to your brain that it's time to unwind and get ready for sleep, making it easier to fall asleep.

Deep Breathing

By simply focusing your attention on your breath, without doing anything to change it, you can prepare your mind and body for rest. It may sound too simple to be useful, but redirecting your thoughts to the natural rhythm of your breath can soothe racing thoughts, relax your body, and help you fall asleep faster. The simplest way to put this into practice is to focus on one area of your body. It could be your stomach rising and falling as you inhale and exhale, or your nostrils as the air passes through them. You could also picture your breath slowly filling

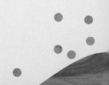

Deep Breathing Techniques

Deep Breathing Techniques

I have found two breathing techniques helpful when I need to relax or distract a busy mind.

Abdominal Breathing

Also called diaphragmatic breathing, this technique is known to increase energy and mental clarity while decreasing stress. While sitting or lying in bed, place your hands on your belly. As you breathe in and out, your hands should rise and fall. Focusing on this movement gets your mind off your busy thoughts and onto your body. It also causes oxygen to enter your bloodstream at the base of your lungs near your diaphragm.

Square Breath

This technique is simple but very effective for distracting a busy mind. While sitting or lying comfortably, breathe in for 4 seconds, picturing a line being drawn, creating the first side of a square. On the exhale, count for 4 seconds and picture the second line of the square. As you inhale, picture the third line for 4 seconds, and on the exhale, imagine the fourth line for 4 seconds. The key is to breathe naturally, without changing your breath—so if 4 seconds is too long or short, choose what works best for you.

and emptying your lungs. Deep breathing techniques can help calm racing thoughts at night and promote feelings of relaxation, especially while you're lying comfortably in bed. The best part is that it's incredibly simple to practice and doesn't take any special skills or tools.

Meditation

Meditation is the process of calming the mind and emotions to experience a state of awareness. It is a simple technique that can be learned in a few minutes and with practice can work instantly to calm racing thoughts and relieve bedtime anxiety. Through the use of meditation and the observation of your thoughts, you develop the power to differentiate between thoughts that are useful and those that are not.

I hear from a lot of people who are eager to try breathing techniques to help with sleep but are averse to trying meditation. The deep breathing techniques above are forms of mindfulness meditation and breath awareness meditation, so you can benefit from applying them without abandoning your belief system.

Progressive relaxation (also referred to as a body scan) is a type of meditation that focuses on finding tension in your body. Typically starting at your toes, you "scan" your body slowly for built-up tension, and then let it go by picturing a release or by physically tensing and relaxing your muscles in that part of your body for a few seconds.

If you find you lose focus or get distracted easily, try repeating positive affirmations instead. You can recite favorite quotes or verses that inspire and encourage you. You might even find yourself reflecting on those words in other moments of your day.

BEDTIME ANXIETY AND RACING THOUGHTS

What does your mind conjure up as you're lying in bed? Are you a worrier? Do you think about what you need to get done at work? Do you contemplate the meaning of life? The biggest sleep obstacles I see again and again are bedtime anxiety and racing thoughts. Our days are busy. Our households are busy. It's no surprise that our brains are active as we fall into bed at night.

Bedtime Anxiety

Whether you have to be up early to catch a flight or give an important presentation at work, keep your evening routine calm and familiar.

Go to bed when you're tired. When tomorrow is a big day, it's natural to want to go to bed early, especially if you need to be up early. If you're a hard-core bedtime thinker, going to bed too soon could result in a lot of lying in bed wide awake, worrying or planning. Changing your bedtime routine can result in throwing off your whole sleep-wake cycle. Treat the night before a big event like any other night and go to bed when you're ready to fall asleep, not when you think you should fall asleep.

Make a to-do list, and then forget about it. If you're afraid you'll forget it, write it down! Make a list of all the things you need to do in the morning, and then put it aside and go to bed knowing that you can take care of everything tomorrow. You should not be lying in bed making lists. Get them out of your head and onto paper so you can sleep soundly. When you start to worry about everything you need to do, tell yourself, "Tomorrow is taken care of, and my only task tonight is to rest."

Don't clock-watch. Set your alarm (even two alarms if you're worried about missing the first one) and turn your digital clocks to face away from you. If you wake up in the middle of the night, don't check the time. It doesn't matter. It will only make you more anxious.

If you wake up prematurely and happen to see the time, think of the sleep you have left as a positive, not a negative. It's a switch you can choose to turn on in your brain to make falling asleep easier. As an example, let's say you go to bed at ten o'clock and you need to be up by six the next morning to leave for the airport. You suddenly wake up at midnight because of noise outside your window. Instead of thinking, "Oh no! I have to be up in six hours!" Change the narrative to "Oh good! I still have six more hours of sleep!" You are choosing the benefit of your remaining sleep over the pressure to fall back to sleep. And if you've learned anything from this book so far, it should be that less stress means more sleep.

Stay positive. Think of all the things that will go well the next day. Picture yourself getting out of bed, finishing your tasks with time to spare, and doing well at whatever job you have to complete. Keep your thoughts light and happy, and if you feel yourself starting to go into a state of worry, tell yourself, "Tomorrow is going to be a great day."

Racing Thoughts

Your thoughts are not the problem that keeps you up at night. Your reaction to those thoughts is the problem. You are allowing your plans and your worries to take over your valuable rest time. When you let go of a thought without reacting, you are taking control and choosing to rest.

The first step is to accept that you have thoughts at bedtime. Your sleep routine includes these thoughts entering your mind.

There is nothing wrong with you, and your thoughts do not have control over you. You are a bedtime thinker.

Next, practice focusing on your breath as you lie in bed. You don't have to do anything fancy, just breathe and think about your breath entering and leaving your nostrils. You can also picture your stomach rising and falling. Keep it simple. When a thought enters your mind, don't fight it and don't entertain it with a reaction. Let it go and return to your breath.

Some people find that speaking to their thoughts helps them let go. Say whatever it is you want to say, or a phrase such as "Not tonight, thank you" or "I'll deal with you tomorrow." Tell your thoughts and worries to leave you alone. Don't let yourself get angry, just say your piece and move on.

Dr. Guy Meadows devotes a whole chapter to mindfulness in *The Sleep Book.* His passion for helping clients deal with negative thoughts has inspired my own practice and love for meditation as a way to calm racing thoughts. You don't have to let your thoughts and worries upset and consume you. They have as much power over you as you allow.

INSOMNIA

I think it's important to know the difference between bedtime anxiety and textbook insomnia because a lot of people consider themselves an "insomniac" without understanding its true meaning. A person who has trouble falling asleep is not

Sleep & Hardship

So what happens when you're knocked off your feet by bad news or a sudden tragedy? When life is tough, we're asked, "How did you sleep last night?" or "Are you sleeping?" We tell each other, "Get some sleep." The ironic part is that sleep is one of the things we need the most, but it's the first thing to suffer when life temporarily falls apart.

Sleep deprivation has never coexisted well with heightened emotions. Sleep should be a priority, but don't be surprised or discouraged if it's a struggle during a difficult time. It can be tough to continue your routine when life has taken an unexpected and unhappy turn. Focus on making bedtime amazingly comforting. Surround yourself with things you love and get in your coziest clothes. Make bedtime a familiar friend as much as possible, so that any negative emotions you start to feel or think then will be unwelcome. Think of going to sleep as confiding in a friend. Speak about it positively. Say to yourself, "I just need some sleep." And "I'll feel better in the morning."

Be kind to yourself and be patient. Take the time you need. Prioritizing sleep won't make your emotions go away, but it will help you handle them. Take care of yourself and know that everything is temporary.

necessarily struggling with insomnia. The definition of insomnia is "difficulty falling asleep and staying asleep, even when a person has the chance to do so," but I believe that definition is missing a key ingredient: the struggle that accompanies not falling asleep. In his book, *The Sleep Solution*, Dr. W. Chris Winter discusses his complete definition of insomnia consisting of two components: a person not sleeping when she wants to sleep, and that the person cares about not sleeping.

An insomniac has trouble falling asleep, and then the stress of not sleeping escalates the problem. To give you an example, a person who can't fall asleep and lies there quietly until they do doesn't have insomnia. A person who can't fall asleep and feels the stress of what will happen if they don't fall asleep is closer to the true diagnosis. There is an inner struggle that accompanies and worsens the problem of not sleeping, and unfortunately, the cycle will inevitably continue. Aside from having difficulty falling asleep, the symptoms of insomnia may include:

- multiple wake-ups during the night
- not feeling well rested in the morning
- daytime sleepiness
- irritability and moodiness
- depression
- general anxiety and anxiety about sleep
- difficulty focusing on tasks

I believe you can experience symptoms of insomnia without being diagnosed with insomnia, as many of the above symptoms are also present with restless sleep, bedtime anxiety, and several sleep disorders.

Whether you suffer from insomnia or symptoms of insomnia, it is important that you consult a professional to find the underlying cause and seek treatment.

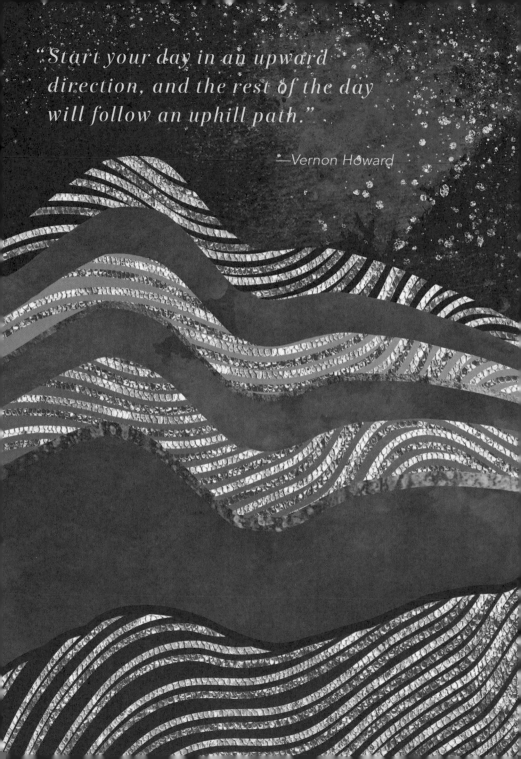

"Start your day in an upward direction, and the rest of the day will follow an uphill path."

—Vernon Howard

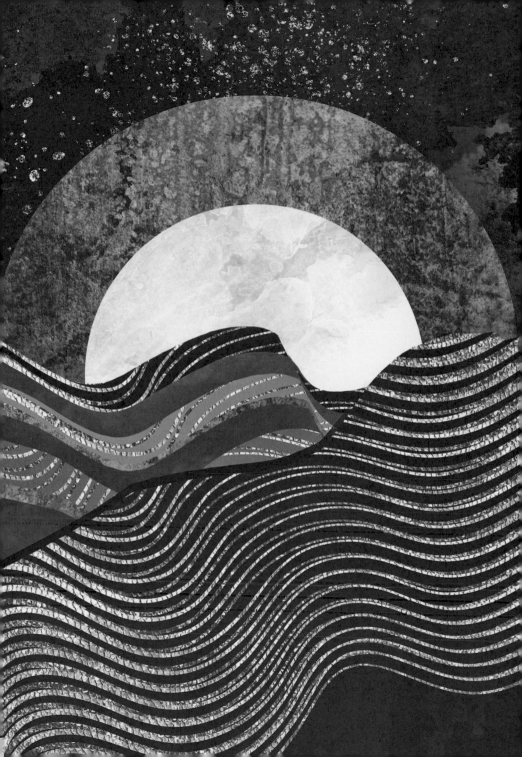

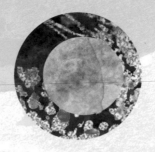

Waking Up

THE SNOOZE BUTTON

It is my hope that you will never use a snooze button again. It has no benefit to you or your sleep whatsoever. When your morning alarm sounds, going back to sleep for a few minutes and waking up, whether it's once or several times, triggers something called "sleep inertia."

Sleep inertia is a transitional state between sleep and wakefulness. It is a state of impaired cognitive performance that occurs immediately after waking, causing prolonged feelings of drowsiness and grogginess. It can take several hours for sleep inertia to dissipate; this means that pressing the snooze button once is choosing nine more minutes of sleep over having a functional first half of the day. Just think of what pressing the snooze button more than once will do.

It's not worth it. If you have time to go back to sleep, you're not using your alarm clock for the reason it was intended. Set a wake-up time and then wake up. Period. Temporarily going back to sleep for a short time will not help you feel less sleepy. It will not help you get out of bed quicker or make waking up easier. Pressing the snooze button is not just prolonging the inevitable, it is making mornings more difficult than they already are.

If you need time to wake up, stay in bed but change your surroundings. Turn on a lamp beside the bed or prop yourself up on a few pillows. Do some light stretches in bed or practice a quick breathing exercise until you feel awake and ready to face the day.

If all else fails, remind yourself that a few minutes of voluntary sleepiness is infinitely better than several hours of miserable drowsiness.

HOW TO BECOME A MORNING PERSON

The term "chronotype" is used to characterize your natural sleep-wake cycle and sleep patterns. In short, it speaks to whether you're a night owl or an early bird or something in between.

A night owl will stay awake until midnight or later and feels energetic just as others are going to bed. Night owls typically have a hard time getting up in the morning and will sleep in or oversleep, given the opportunity. An early bird person rises with the sun and prefers to start the day then because that's when they feel most active and creative.

There are four general chronotypes and each one refers to a different pattern of sleep-wake cycles:

Bears sleep and wake according to the sun, feeling most active during the day and sleepy at night. They feel most productive midmorning and experience an energy dip as a midafternoon slump.

Wolves (night owls) fall asleep later and wake up later. They get their energy in the middle of the day and the evening when others are winding down. Night owls tend to sleep on the weekends to try to make up for the sleep debt they accumulate during the workweek.

Lions (early birds) wake up early and are most productive in the morning. They get most of their essential tasks done before noon, feel naturally sleepy by early evening, and are often in bed before everyone else.

Dolphins are most productive from midmorning to the early afternoon. They have a harder time staying asleep at night, making it difficult for them to follow a regular sleep routine.

Each chronotype has its benefits, and one is not inherently better than the others. Your chronotype is based on your biology and genetic makeup.

I want to challenge the idea that you are stuck with the chronotype you have been born with, if and when you feel it is no longer serving you. My experiment might have worked because of my age, but I have switched from being a wolf to a lion over the past few years and I am happier for it.

As a teenager, I was a night owl who rarely went to bed before midnight. If that sounds like every teenager you've ever known, that's because puberty sparks a shift in the sleep-wake cycle. For teenagers, melatonin is released much later in the evening, delaying feelings of sleepiness. The result is falling asleep late at night and having a hard time waking up for class at 8 a.m.

In my twenties and most of my thirties, I was a night owl because the evening was my only free time to work on creative projects. Sure, I was tired at 2 a.m., but there was no way I was going to abandon the design I was working on to lie in bed and think about the project for at least another hour. I was frequently going to bed in the wee hours of the morning, then dragging myself out of bed the next morning to go to my full-time job.

Was I a true night owl during those years, feeling energetic in the evening while everyone else was asleep, or was I forcing myself to take advantage of the only hours I believed I had to be productive? I don't know, but I wouldn't say it was working for me.

In my late thirties, at a time when I was finally happy in my full-time nine-to-five work, I felt an ache to start my own business. I was always working on a side hustle as an adult, and my entrepreneurial genes longed for a creative outlet, but I had no available time or energy. I had to make a change in my schedule and sleep habits if I wanted to work on my new venture, and I had one viable option. I had to become one of those annoying morning people.

My experiment was gradual. I would wake up an hour earlier and work on my website design. Then when I realized I needed more time for creating content, I would wake up two hours earlier. As time passed and I had more blog posts to write and more podcasts to record, I was waking up a little earlier and easier every time. I was motivated and excited about my work, and that made my early mornings less torturous.

Even so, to this day I still wake up every morning wanting to go back to sleep. I don't like getting out of bed and I never have. Becoming a functional morning person has been an ongoing choice. In all fairness, my age has probably helped my ability to wake up earlier. A lot of people find that as they get older, they turn into early birds. I'm not ancient, but I am approaching middle age.

Consider another explanation for not liking mornings. I have realized, after finally getting my sleep habits in order, that wanting to stay in bed every morning doesn't mean I slept poorly and need more sleep. It means I like my bed, something I openly admit, and my alarm is probably waking me up in the middle of a deep sleep.

Dreams happen during REM sleep, so if you're waking up aware that you were dreaming, you were in in this phase of sleep. Having your deep and REM sleep stages disrupted by an alarm can leave you feeling sleepy and groggy for several minutes. I tell you this to let you know that not everybody springs out of bed in the morning and happily belts out "Good morning, Baltimore" like Tracy Turnblad in *Hairspray*. You might not wake up twirling with cartoon birds on your arms like Cinderella, and it doesn't necessarily mean you're sleep-deprived. It's okay if it takes you some time to get going in the morning.

If you are sleepy all the time no matter how much sleep you get at night, it can be helpful to see your doctor and ask to have a sleep test done.

CREATING AN ENJOYABLE MORNING ROUTINE

In the same way an evening routine can help you transition into sleep, an enjoyable morning routine can help you feel more awake and ready to start your day. If you have a project you've been dreaming of designing or you want more time to pursue your interests undisturbed, here are some ways you can take advantage of the pure magic of a morning routine:

Change your alarm. Place your alarm clock across the room from your bed, so you're forced to get up and turn it off. If you're already out of bed and walking around, it will be easier to stay up. Change your alarm to a sound that doesn't make you want to throw it against a wall. Download a song that makes you happy or choose a ringtone that makes you want to dance. You may want to download a smartphone app that vibrates to gradually wake you up. Similarly, a sunlight alarm clock will glow in steady intervals to wake you without suddenly ripping you from a deep sleep. People who use these types of alarm clocks say that they feel less drowsy upon waking.

Make your bed. It's harder to get back into bed when it's already made. It's even harder when the sheets are tucked in and the decorative pillows are in place. And as I wrote earlier, you'll feel as if you've already accomplished something.

Let the sunlight in. In the first few moments after you wake up and make your bed, open the curtains to let the light into your room and your home.

Exposure to sunlight releases serotonin in the brain, contributing to well-being, enhanced mood, and lower levels of stress. Sunlight reduces melatonin levels, helping you feel more alert and awake.

Move your body. If you naturally feel energetic in the morning, it's an excellent time for a workout. If exercising is the last thing you want to do when you first get out of bed, try doing some slow movements that increase your heart rate without exerting too much energy. Practices such as yoga, stretching, and walking can lower cortisol levels and blood pressure and improve your mood.

Schedule something special. What do you need more of in your life right now? Schedule it into your morning routine. If you're craving some alone time, the morning can be incredibly peaceful. If you're looking for time to spend on a creative project, take advantage of the boost in imagination and energy your brain may experience during the early hours. If you're looking for a quiet moment to enjoy your coffee while you read a novel, fill your favorite mug and go for it.

Design a morning routine that inspires and delights you, and you'll set the intention for your entire day. Your morning can be rushed and stressful or it can be calm and enjoyable. It's entirely up to you.

Conclusion

Making sleep a priority is the ultimate act of self-care and self-love. By working with your internal body clock, you are embracing the science of sleep and its endless health benefits. When you start yawning in the evening, consider it a cue to start getting ready for bed, as you look forward to a calm and cozy night of sleep. This is the perfect time to decide what life you want to wake up to tomorrow. Nobody sleeps perfectly every night, but you have more control than you think. The way you speak, the way you think, and the small choices you make today will have a profound impact on your sleep tonight.

So what do you need more of in your life right now? I can pretty much guarantee that whatever it is, sleep can help with that.

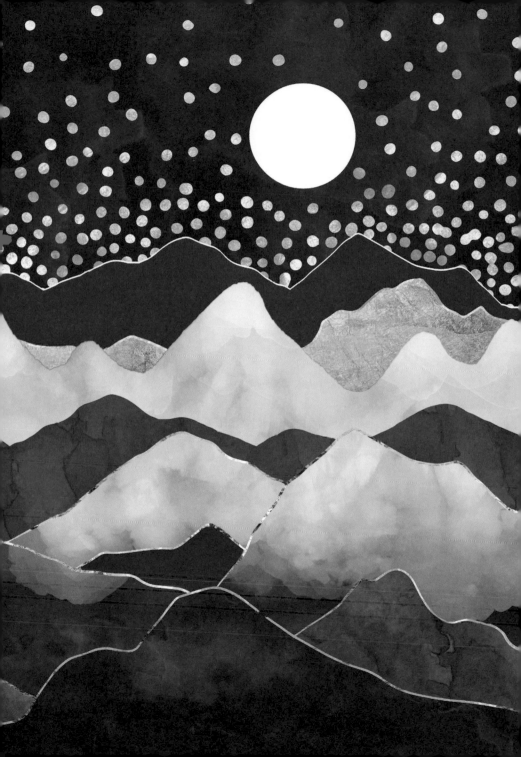

Resources

Books

Fast Asleep, Wide Awake by Dr. Nerina Ramlakhan
Sleep by Nick Littlehales
The Sleep Book Dr. Guy Meadows
Sleep Smarter by Shawn Stevenson
The Sleep Solution by W. Chris Winter, MD
Wide Awake and Dreaming by Julie Flygare

Websites

CPAPBabes (cpapbabes.com)
Hypersomnia Foundation (hypersomniafoundation.org)
Julie Flygare (julieflygare.com)
National Sleep Foundation (sleepfoundation.org)
Project Sleep (project-sleep.com)

Sleep Aids

Endy® Weighted Blanket (ca.endy.com)
Flare Audio Sleeep® earplugs (flareaudio.com)
Manta Sleep Mask (mantasleep.com)
Plant Therapy® essential oils (planttherapy.com)
Sleep Crown™ over-the-head pillow (sleepcrown.com)
SleepPhones® sleep headphones (sleepphones.com)
Somnifix® Strips (somnifix.com)
Sound Oasis® Sleep Sound Therapy Systems (soundoasis.com)
TrueDark® glasses (truedark.com)

Acknowledgments

To my Dad, author Daniel Wyatt. I can't believe he did this ten times while raising a family and working full time. He's been an amazing example of making space in your busy life for whatever you're passionate about. And he was a great dad at the same time. Thank you for being a phone call away.

To my Mom, my biggest fan. For decades, she has been telling me, "There are people out there who are less talented than you who are successful at what you want to do." When I needed to hear it, she would add, "The only difference between them and you is that they're doing it." (Ouch! But true.) This advice has helped me overcome my own self-doubt. A handful of years ago, she told me to pick one thing I wanted to do and focus on it. So, I picked online coaching. If it weren't for her advice, I would be running two Etsy shops, with four different small businesses registered under my name, and selling fermented food out of the back of a van. Thank you for being my mom, friend, and mentor. I hope your mango's ripe.

To my brother, Barrie. My opposite in so many ways, but also my first friend and partner-in-crime. When I was a baby he wanted me to move away. Now our relationship is based on a series of inside jokes and quotes from '90s sitcoms. Barrie didn't buy a copy of my book because he thought he was getting one for free. He was right.

To Jake Lowe, my life partner, hero, and best friend. He's been lovingly supporting all of my bad business ideas, and haircuts, since 2005. Knowing he's proud of me and hearing him brag about my book gives me goosebumps. Choosing him was my life's other great accomplishment.

To Marnie, my favorite friend since childhood. She knew how exciting getting a book deal was for me and didn't disappoint with her reaction to the news. There are too many things to say about a ride-or-die friend to list here, so I'll simply say thank you. Here's to another thirty years of laughing till we can't breathe.

To my brother-in-law, Kevin Lowe. He is still my favorite person to crochet winter woollies for. Thanks for being a constant cheerleader over text message through this whole process.

To the incredible team at Quarto who worked so hard to get this book published, particularly through a global pandemic. We should have a dance party once we're all allowed to be in the same room together. To my publisher, Rage Kindelsperger, for finding me on Instagram and believing I could write an interesting book on sleep. I'm so relieved I didn't delete her DM after thinking it was spam. To Erin Canning, my editor and my main contact over the past year. I believe she did a happy dance with me the day the book proposal was approved. Her morning emails brought me either good news or more homework, but her patience and humor made the process fun. To Laura Drew, Jen Cogliantry, and SpaceFrog Designs: Thanks for designing a beautiful book with a cover that I am still planning to somehow tattoo on my entire body. To Todd Conley, my marketing manager: Thanks for making me sound cool enough on paper for strangers to want to interview me.

To Lori Kennedy, my kickass business coach. Without her no-bullshit guidance, I would still be a struggling general wellness coach, tweaking my website design daily, and wondering why no one wants to work with me.

To my business besties, April and Sandy, for celebrating with me every time I came up with another boring idea for a lead magnet. They have made the entrepreneurship journey less lonely. Thanks for being my people.

To Rae Connell, for taking my author photo. We might have to do another portrait session soon because I cut my hair again. To Melika Sharifi, for making me photo ready. You made me look like a grown-ass professional woman. You are magic.

To Zac Lowe, for helping me with the bedroom plant section of this book. Sorry for killing your plants while you were away on vacation.

To my all-time favorite teacher, Gary DaCosta, for making high school bearable. He believed my smart-ass class projects might one day lead to a positive contribution to society, and I'm hoping this book is it. Otherwise, I'm open to suggestions.